PLANT BASED DIET COOKBOOK FOR BEGINNERS

Plant based diet cookbook for beginners: 300 healthy and tasty plant-based recipes for a vegetarian lifestyle. 21 days Meal plan Included.

Table of Contents

Introduction

A Plant-based diet is any dieting plan that is designed to accommodate only foods that are derived from plant sources. Typically, plant sources for a plant-based diet include grains, nuts, seeds, vegetables, legumes, and fruits.

Different people have a different perception of what a plant-based diet should be, and this, in part, stands as the reason why most people (flexitarian still include a small number of animal products such as fish and meat while feeding mainly on vegetarian foods. However, another group of people (pescatarian still practice a plant-based diet lifestyle that cut out meat but still including fish. On the other hand, other groups of plant-based dieters (vegetarian forbid meat, fish but still welcome eggs and other dairy products.

Generally, it is observed that people following a plant-based diet consume a wide range of vegetables, fruits as well as pulses. With this, they are most likely to have a good intake of vitamins, dietary fibers, minerals, potassium, and folate, which are present in vegetables and fruits and are essential for a healthy living.

When considering what is deemed as non-processed, remember that these are natural foods that are whole, unrefined, or with minimally refined ingredients.

As you go through your search, remember that it is all about feeling better and getting control over how food affects your body. Hence, focusing on the different tasty groups that you will be enjoying is where you should start!

Thus, when it comes to your produce, people may say that "fresh is best." It does require some research for your area because sometimes, it may not be the best option available for a number of reasons.

There are numerous things influencing the nutrients that your produce contains. The harvest date and time, the proximity of source, and the duration of the display are just some of the important fluctuating circumstances. Some others are the duration of their contact with light as well as the temperature at which they are stored. These factors have the capability to impact the nutrition extractible from these produce drastically. Now, in the huge stores wherein people typically buy their products, the general public does not have knowledge of the aforementioned factors. Moreover, considering the technology today, personally evaluating the quality of the said produce is not so simple anymore, no matter how hard you try. Hence, if it is in your power to do so, opt to purchase from small but credible sources whose methods of product acquisition are known to you. Only by then that you can try getting the best you can for your dollar.

However, let's not forget that a cost-effective way of buying produce exists through your local freezer section. It is also beneficial at times that you don't have the time to prepare food. One fact that might interest you is that the nutrients of frozen produce are relatively high. This is largely due to the fact that they are on prime condition during the time that they are taken. You can take advantage of frozen produce for out-of-season items, However, always keep in mind that like anything else, its nutritional quality still depreciates as time passes by. Hence, immediate consumption is still advised.

When you go to buy breakfast cereal, almond milk, bread (whole grain), hot sauce, and pasta, make it your habit to see its list of contents in advance—the less the contents, the better. As an example, pasta completely composed of whole grain wheat and preservative-free bread can be an option, as long as they don't have any animal products (meat by-products, dairy, or egg). If it's grain-based, check its authenticity (in terms of its actual composition). A good rule of thumb is that if the term "whole" isn't explicitly indicated, then it is most likely refined, and it's better to pass that option up.

In our ventures down the grocery aisle, picking through different products, we want also to pay attention to added salt. Usually, there's a lot of them that can be found especially from packaged items. Generally speaking, for the Plant-Based Diet to be successful, a daily sodium consumption of 1500 mg must be the maximum. To do this successfully, you shouldn't completely rely on the percentages indicated, as 2300 mg is the typically suggested intake of the said element that they use.

And finally, when reading labels, we want to make sure that you are not consuming refined sugar. There are multiple names for added sugar, so understanding what they are is important. While there may be very small amounts of added sweeteners to many of the things we may use off the shelf, the focus is to eliminate as much as possible. The more you read, the more you will learn about certain brands and their content. However, in the beginning, don't worry too much, and do the best that you can. Something to also keep in mind in your choice is the existence of various sugar classifications, which may be really far down the ingredient list.

As you have seen, there are a lot of different aspects of this diet to consider as you start the process. The key is to keep it as simple as possible for you and your lifestyle because the point is: you want to be successful and not burdened down.

Hence, when you move through this book, remember that it is all about you being in control.

Here are the FOUR main groups that you will be building your meals from:

WHOLE GRAINS – These are food products made from whole or complete grains that contain the three key parts of a seed: the bran, germ, and endosperm. Some of these are bread, cereals, pasta, brown rice, quinoa, millet, oats, barley, corn, and bulgur. The bonus of whole grain foods is that they are very filling—without the fat!

The good news about this group is that research has shown that in countries where these grains are a staple, some diseases such as diabetes, heart disease, and cancer are much less common. They are filled with important nutrients including protein, fiber, B vitamins, antioxidants, iron, zinc, copper, and magnesium, or trace minerals.

LEGUMES – These are plants that bear fruit that grow in pods which can be broken down into different subsections including beans, lentils, peas, and peanuts. Some very familiar legumes are chickpeas (also known as garbanzo beans), kidney beans, black beans, soybeans, pinto beans, and navy beans. These hearty, high protein foods are rich in calcium, iron, cholesterol-lowering soluble fiber, and even traces of omega 3 fatty acids.

FRUITS AND VEGETABLES – The obvious base of this diet that is loaded with vitamins and minerals, and is very low in fat. Like all plant foods and tubers (root vegetables), they have no cholesterol at all. For the most part, fruits and vegetables are lower in calories than many other foods, so choosing to eat more, can help to lower your overall daily calorie count.

One great thing to do is to become aware of different kinds of vegetables and fruits that you might not have been familiar with. When you do this, you really help to expand your produce horizons. This book will help you learn how to prepare them properly too. The goal being, you may have thought you didn't like a particular veggie, but making it a new way could completely change how you feel!

A great benefit of eating whole fruits and vegetables adds fiber to your diet, which fills you up and helps you maintain your weight. An added bonus is, with a variety of colors, flavors, and textures; it brings life to meals and snacks. For example, you can start eating fruit for a snack instead of cookies and/or chips. By steadily adding plant-based foods into your diet, you'll be getting your mind and body used to enjoying them!

NUTS AND SEEDS – These foods may be small but are nutrient and energy-packed—loaded with vitamins, minerals, fiber, protein, and essential fatty acids such as Omega 3 fatty acids. This nutrient is a great anti-inflammatory and great for the health of our brain, skin, hair and hormone production. Adding them to meals, snacks, and desserts makes this versatile food a great addition to a healthier eating routine.

In our recipe chapters, you will learn how easy it is to create tasty and easy meals full of these categories and more. You can have full control in replacing your tastes and habits to change your health for the better. Don't feel you have to put a time table on disentangling yourself from the behaviors and patterns you have had your whole eating life. Expect to find foods you enjoy and new methods in shopping and cooking. You will love it when this becomes your new normal!

Plant-Based Whole Food Quick Reference

•Legumes

•navy beans, peas, lentils, etc.

•Leaves

•lettuce, spinach, arugula, etc.

•Bulbs

•onion, garlic, shallots, etc.

•Roots

•beet, potato, carrot, etc.

•Flowers

•cauliflower, broccoli, etc.

•Whole Grains

•wheat, brown rice, rye, etc.

•Fruits

•tomato, orange, kiwi, etc.

•Mushrooms

•Portobello, button, shiitake, etc.

•Stems

•celery, rhubarb, asparagus, etc.

•Nuts

•almonds, walnuts, sunflower seeds, etc.

Animal-Based Food Products Quick Reference

•Dairy

•cheese, milk, yogurt, butter, etc.

•Eggs

•chicken eggs, duck eggs, etc.

•Fish & Seafood

•tuna, swordfish, shrimp, scallops, clams, etc.

•Meat

•beef, pork, lard, etc.

•Poultry

•chicken, turkey, quail, duck, etc.

Chapter 1. Benefits of The Plant Based Diet

It is essential to understand that a plant-based meal plan does not necessarily mean permanently eliminating animal products from your diet. It involves incorporating more and more plants and vegetables in your diet. It is a way of eating to satisfaction while not denying your body the essential nutrients it requires. Perception is in mind. Therefore, before one decides to stick to a plant-based meal, it is imperative to feed in your thinking that it is the best for your body, mind, and soul. That way, you'll start developing taste and liking for the plant-based meal, and with time, you will find it sweet and very fulfilling.

A plant-based meal has been used over the years both for therapeutic or just nutritional value. There are some vegetables which you may not find tasty, delicious, or sweet. The bitter plant adding fresh herb seasoning, and some can even be blended when making a smoothie. Always try to make it in a way that you can comfortably consume because sometimes it's not very sweet to the mouth but very good to the body.

If we eat a lot of plants, it means we are getting vitamins, fiber, and phytochemicals. These are nutrients that our bodies fall short of, thus keeping us away from taking a lot of supplements. While vegan meal emphasizes strictly eating plant-based food and zero animal product, plant-based meal incorporates animal protein but in minimal quantity. Plant-based meal thus is very accommodative and less restricting thus creates smooth and easy transitioning when one decides to start.

• A lot of emphasis on whole foods and minimal focus on processed food. Always Whole foods mainly are Plant-based while processed food mostly comprises of animal products. A plant-based diet is high in nutrients and contains fewer calories. For this reason, even when taken in large quantities, it's not easy for someone to gain weight compared to processed foods. The ease in absorption and digestion and the extra fiber helps prevent constipation.

• Focuses mostly on the plant, which includes but not limited to fruits, whole grains, vegetables, legumes, nuts, seeds, and vegetables. These should comprise the majority of the food one eats, and one should very strict enough to follow the diet. All serving should contain more plants and less animal protein to enjoy the full benefits.

• Quality is more important than quantity; by this, I mean fresh, locally available, or organic is healthier and nutritious. You can liaise with local farmers and get fresh farm produce and prepare at home. Fresh from the farm is more nutritious and very tasty. Green vegetables lose their nutrients with time if not appropriately stored; thus should be cooked while still green.

• Always consume fats that are healthy, avoid refined fats and oil processed with lots of chemicals. Go for unsaturated fats, which are very good and healthy for your heart. Unhealthy fats are hard to absorb and sometimes bring some health risks like blocked arteries and diabetes.

• Start your plant-based with breakfast because this is the meal no one would think should have any vegetables at all. You can take fruit salad; add spinach or kale to your eggs or cauliflower smoothie. Healthy breakfast every morning is crucial and should be taken with seriousness, especially if one has started a vegetarian diet. It will give your body the energy needed to start and go through the day, thus making your brain active throughout the day.

- Experiment with at least one plant every week. It will increase the variety of vegetables you're used to every week. Additionally, it will also boost your nutrient every week but also make you have a variety to choose from, thus reducing restrictions. It will also expose you to a big world of the various plant-based meal and categorize them as in, easy to prepare, favorite, most nutritious, and tastier.

Health Benefits of a Plant-Based Meal

Reduce Risk of Obesity

Across the globe, millions of people are struggling with obesity or weight-related issues. Sometimes it may be due to eating habits, lifestyle, or genetics. Today, people have not succeeded in losing weight. Striving for a realistic exercise routine is crucial as compared to diet pills, which are very harmful to the body.

Clinical research has shown that a more plant-based diet can help decrease obesity, promoting healthy weight loss. A vegan and vegetarian lifestyle has a significantly low risk of obesity or overweight. Plant-based diet often has high fiber, which is good for digestion and prevents constipation. This helps clear the digestive tract, thus raising the body's metabolism. A plant-based diet is a very healthy way to lose weight without worrying so much about your body, not getting the necessary nutrients. It is also important to note; not all vegetarian diets are healthy.

Obesity can cause many health-related complications and in severe cases, can even hinder morbidity. So whether you want to lose weight for health reasons or to keep fit then Plant-based meal is the best option. If you compare the room food needs in your stomach, you'll realize Plant-based meal takes less space. Thus you'll consume fewer calories.

Reduce Cancer Risk

Cancer cannot be cured by eating a plant-based diet. It will help reduce one's chances of acquiring cancer, but it must go along with healthy habits and behaviors. Some of these healthy behaviors include alcohol limit, exercise, maintaining a body weight that is normal according to one's body mass index (BMI).

A plant-based diet can help prevent a significant percentage of cancer cases if it can at least prevent then it is a dietary habit worth emulating. The plant-based meal diet should have lots of fruits, beans, nuts, seeds, and grains with some limited animal food that can prevent cancer. Those kinds of diets contain fiber, minerals, and vitamins that hinder the growth of cancerous cells.

Foods to avoid include but not limited to: fast foods like cheeseburgers, sausages, French fries, chicken nuggets, and hot dogs; refined sugar, canned foods, added sugar, artificial sweetener, and processed animal foods. The phytochemical available in plant-based meals can fight and thwart cancer cells. It is, therefore, essential to replace unhealthy food with plant-based meals to lead a healthy and more fulfilling life.

Cancer is now a global problem affecting both children and adults, impoverished and wealthy alike, and the cost of treating cancer can drain a family's financial resources. Sometimes, crowdfunding needs to be done to raise the required money for treatment. It is thus essential to adopt the habit of eating a plant-based meal and form it to be part of you until your system gets used to it.

Start with the plant you are familiar with and are locally available in your area. Then as you make it, routinely try new healthy plant-based recipes, and if you work during lunch, consider packing your lunch from home. Processed and unhealthy food in the diet may rapidly increase the growth of cancer cells for cancer patients. Plant-based meals can also be used as a detox, especially when blended. This applies to fruits and vegetables that can be eaten raw.

Low Risk of Heart Disease

Most plant-based meals are heart-healthy in that they favor the general functioning of the earth. Plant-based meals reduce the risk of developing heart-related diseases like high or low blood pressure, heart attack, and liver problems. We need to note, however, that the quality of the foods consumed and the types matter a lot. This is because high-quality nutrients have the necessary nutrients needed for organ functioning, thus making it practical and healthy.

The heart is the central circulatory system, it is responsible for adding oxygen in the blood, then pumping it throughout the body, and when it stops, then one dies. Not all but various heart diseases are associated with unhealthy eating habits, overconsumption of processed food, and lack of exercise. This diet involves eating food with fewer fats. The advantage of this is that it promotes a healthy heart, which can, in turn, lead to a healthy lifestyle. So most cardiovascular diseases can be prevented by adopting a plant-based meal plan.

Low Risk of Type 2 Diabetes

A plant-based meal does not only reduce the risk of getting type two diabetes, but it can also be a very effective way of managing diabetes. Studies have shown that there is a high prevalence of type two diabetes concerning eating patterns consisting of mainly processed food, animal protein, and refined sugars.

A plant-based meal has potential benefits since it improves the resistance of insulin in the body, promoting recommended and healthy body weight. Increased fiber improves food interactions while decreasing the amount of saturated fat in the body. Those who love eating meat are twice likely at risk of having diabetes later in life as compared to those who eat more plants or vegetarians. Plant-based meals contain significantly insulin sensitivity that is high, which is crucial in maintaining the recommended sugar level that is healthy.

Improved Digestion

Digestion of food is essential because it determines absorption. Plan based meal is naturally packed with fiber, which is key to proper and better digestion. Fiber brings additional bulk to one's stool while assisting in regulating, thus smooth elimination of undigested food and stool. When absorption is adequate, the body feels functional and active as well as the need is involved in various activities throughout the day.

When digestion is proper, there is reduced discomfort associated with problems arising from indigestion, overeating, and eating fatty foods that stay longer in the stomach and take longer to digest and absorb. This will mean the necessary and healthy nutrients are easily absorbed in the bloodstream and the wastes comfortably removed without discomfort or pain. Drinking a lot of water as recommended, also eases digestion.

Boost Energy Naturally

Plant-based meals are very rich in minerals and vitamins, which give people a lot of energy. The nutrients also act as antioxidants, and the healthy protein and fats boost brain functioning and make one alert. A plant-based meal is easy to digest and has that extra energy that they release to the body, which enables the body to be more active and boost thinking and improves mood. This is the reason why most professional athletes love and prefer plant-based meals.

Fast foods take longer to digest, slows metabolism, and leaves the body weak and inactive, thus can lead to unnecessary weight gain. Natural energy is more effective than energy derived from energy drinks since it is coming due to satisfaction and not an instant boost. Thus it is essential for everyone, not just athletes, to consume lots of plant proteins so that they can have natural energy to carry out daily tasks.

Healthy Hair, Skin, & Nails

This may sound absurd, but it's true; your hair, skin, and nails are most of the time 90%your diet. What you feed your body and go inside your body will be reflected outside. The vitamins and minerals are good for skin, smoothens skin, repairs dead cells as well as give the skin room to breathe.

Meat and dairy products can cause inflammation, which will be visible in the skin. But to achieve the smooth surface, be consistent with your plant-based diet, and be patient because the change will not be realized immediately but after a very long time. Skin can also appear hydrated and not dry; this is a sign of more plant-based meals in the diet.

Plant-Based Meals & Your Health

Those who love meat and fast food often struggle when they start a plant-based diet and can sometimes even find it annoying. Doctors will recommend reducing animal protein intake and maximizing on plants, but how many times have we ignored doctors' recommendations? It's not comfortable with the current fast-paced life, which gives no time to prepare a home-cooked meal.

Also, some people stay places far away from farmers or where access to fresh farm produce is not easy; however, there are some tips you can use so that you don't run out of stock and start indulging. You can buy groceries in bulk worth one week and ensure you store them properly. Poor storage can spoil them, thus making them not suitable for human consumption.

Compared to fast and processed food, Plant-based meals can be slightly expensive, that's why some people may be tempted to grab fast food during lunch, which is cheaper and readily available. It is thus useful to look at long term benefits, potential risks, and your state of health. The cost of medication is or maybe even more expensive than plants and vegetables. This long term benefit makes it worth investing in plant-based meals, which are fresh, nutritious, and healthy.

Kindly keep in mind that people who have some of the diseases discussed above are not vegetarian, and this plant-based meal will not prevent one from getting those diseases, but the diet lowers the risk. Your doctor needs to give you consent if you're on medication or if you have some allergies or just for the doctor to provide you with the approval that it's okay to start a plant-based meal.

Some people are allergic to some grains or nuts; you can get an alternative that is healthy and has the same of better nutritional value. The plant should be included from the first meal of the day, which is breakfast. Include as much as you possibly can, make it appetizing and appealing, if you don't know where to start from do not worry since the next chapters have some simple yet effective recipes that you can use. The recipes contain breakfast, lunch, and supper.

If you are doing a plant-based meal for health reasons, bring your family on board if possible, let them know why you have decided to change your eating habit. Chances are, they will be very appreciative and would give the necessary moral support that you need, you'll also be helping them as they will also consume healthy plant meals, thus live healthier fulfilling lives.

Family and friends can also give recommendations on where to get fresh produce; they can motivate and encourage one another. Eating plant-based meals will help you realize a healthy lifestyle. Thus healthy living; people who live healthy lives, have more fulfilling, and rewarding lives, therefore, they are happier content, and less anxious. They are also active and not conscious of their bodies since they are rarely overweight.

Not all plant-based meal is healthy the same way as not all animal protein is harmful. So as you embark on a plant-based meal, confirm and recheck the quality and nutritional values. The best part about a plant-based diet is the low-calorie rate and less fatty. Ensure that you take the recommended calories without overindulging or depriving yourself.

The best news with a plant-based diet is you are not permanently restricted from taking animal protein, but you can choose it in very minimal quantities. This is good news for animal protein lovers and makes the meal plan workable and worth trying. The diet is also progressive in the sense that you can start slowly and not necessarily cutting on all animal protein intake at ago.

Health workers are currently encouraging people who are not sick to east healthy so as to boost their immunity and help their body be able to fight some pathogens without medication. It is also interesting to note that medicines are made using herbs and some plants. Why wait to be sick if a plant-based meal can prevent some sicknesses?

Plant-based meal, therefore, is an essential diet, and if everyone can get started, then we can have a very healthier nation. It is one of the most inclusive vegetarian related diets. Different places have different plants depending on the season so you can take advantage of the season and purchase fresh and locally produced and enjoy the raw nutrients.

Also, one can link with local farmers and ensure that you get quality for your money or instead of purchasing immediately it's got from the farm and prepare the same day, thus preserving the nutrients. A plant-based meal is not easy but realistic and doable as long as you put your mind to it. Redefine yourself today and start consuming a plant-based diet.

Chapter 2. Shopping List

Shopping for a plant-based diet plan sounds tough, but it is pretty much easier. We are providing you with a list of foods that you can opt for while following the diet plan. You don't need to stick solely to this list; rather we recommend making changes to make the diet plan more versatile. The only thing to keep in mind is that it should be having plant-based ingredients. One more important thing to understand is that the formulation of products might change, so you have to keep a close eye on the labels on foods. The list includes the following:

1.Fresh Produce (Veggies and Fruits

You can have a wide variety of fresh vegetables and fruits. Go for various dark leafy green veggies. We recommend avoiding avocados if you have cardiac complications and eat more if you are aiming to lose weight.

2.Legumes and Beans

You can enjoy all variants of lentils and dried beans. In case you opt for canned beans, prefer going for no salt or low-sodium. If you are unable to find any no-salt-added beans, rinse the beans thoroughly before using them.

3.Seeds, Nuts, and Dried Fruits

Don't go for nuts if you have cardiac complications and eat more of them if you wish to lose weight. In case you opt for nuts, every variant is better but prefer going for no-oil added or raw. Don't eat them by the handful as their fat content is high, and so is their calorie content, and it can make you overeat it. You can also use nut butter.

You can go for omega-3 rich flax and chia seeds for topping cereals and even replacing eggs in your baking recipes. The content should be 1 tbsp. of chia or ground flaxseed in addition to 3 tbsp of water, which is the equivalent of 1 egg. Whole flax seeds are hard to digest, so prefer going for ground flaxseed, or you can grind them in a coffee grinder before usage. Eat more seeds like pumpkin seeds, sesame, and sunflower seeds, etc.

Go for dried fruits, but keep in mind that they are not having any added sugar. One more important thing to remember is that that are having higher calories than fresh fruits. If you have a diabetic condition or are aiming to lose weight, prefer going for fresh fruits instead of dried ones. Moreover, avoid having dried banana chips as they are fried most of the time.

4.Frozen Fruits

You can have all types of frozen veggies and fruits without having dairy ingredients or added oil.

5.Bread

Prefer going for bread that is prepared from 100 percent whole grain and does not have any oil added or have more than 10 percent of calorie content credited to fats. Don't go for unbleached wheat flour, organic wheat flour. Enriched wheat flour and wheat flour are not whole grain-based flours. You can use the following:

•Rudi's Organic Bakery 100% Whole Wheat (not 100% oil-free but very low-fat

•Trader Joe's Whole Wheat Tuscan Pane (double-check it is the whole wheat variety

•Food for Life Ezekiel 4:9 breads, English muffins, and tortillas

•Engine 2 Tortillas (Whole Foods

•Dave's Killer Bread

•Trader Joe's Corn and Wheat Tortillas

6.Whole Grains

You can have a wide variety of whole grains in your diet plan i.e. rice, spelt, millet, whole-grain polenta, quinoa, bulgur, farro, hull-less barley, teff, oatmeal, and many more.

You can also have a wide variety of whole-grain rice like long, medium, and short-grain, black, red, purple, wild, jasmine, and much more. You can have any type of rice, but not white rice on the plant-based diet plan.

You can have a wide array of whole-grain flours in your diet plan too. These include:

•Whole wheat pastry flour

•White whole wheat flour

•Whole wheat flour

•Oat Flour

•Barley Flour

•Amaranth Flour

•Rye Flour

•Spelt Flour

•Kamut Flour

Apart from these, you can also go for gluten-free flours if you are having any allergies to wheat. But it is important to read the labels carefully as various gluten-free flours are processed.

7.Pasta

You are allowed to have any 100 percent whole wheat or brown rice pasta. You can also go for other pasta made from quinoa, spelt, etc. but you have to ensure that it is 100 percent whole grain.

8.Breakfast Cereals

You can choose any whole grain hot or cold minimally sweetened cereals, which is not having any added oils. For convenience, see the following:

•Steel Cut Oatmeal

•Original Cheerios

•Grape Nuts

•Rolled (Old FashionedOats

•Bran Flakes

•Wheat Chex

•Engine 2 Cereals and Granola

•Non-Dairy "Milks"

You can also go for either minimally sweetened or unsweetened non-dairy beverages too. You should also avoid having products that are having any oil in their ingredients. You should also avoid oat non-dairy beverages because of its sugar content. You can have the following:

•Almond Breeze Original Unsweetened or Vanilla Unsweetened

•Wegmans Organic Original Soymilk, Unsweetened

•Trader Joe's Organic Soy Beverage Unsweetened

•Wegmans Almond Beverage, Original Unsweetened and Vanilla Unsweetened

•Trader Joe's Almond Beverage, Original Unsweetened and Vanilla Unsweetened

•Engine 2 Almond milk

•Silk Unsweetened Cashew milk

•Silk Unsweetened Original or Unsweetened Vanilla Almond milk

•Engine 2 Almond milk

9.Pasta and Tomato Sauces

You should go for sauces having 10 percent or lesser calories from fat, or no animal products or no added oil, or minimal sugar, and lower sodium content when you are comparing these products.

10.Salad Dressings (Prepared

You should go for dressings having 10 percent or lesser calories from fat, or no animal products or no added oil, or minimal sugar, and lower sodium content when you are comparing these products.

11.Flavor Boosters

You can have various flavor boosters to enhance the flavor of your food without the addition of any sugar or fat. These flavor boosters include:

Vinegar: White balsamic, balsamic, flavored balsamic, white wine vinegar, apple cider vinegar, unseasoned rice vinegar, and many more.

Herbs and Spices: Ginger and garlic (minced or fresh in jars without having added sodium), fresh herbs, individual spices, and other sodium flavor blends, etc.

Mustards: You are not allowed to have high sugar honey mustard sauces.

Capers: You should rinse it before usage for minimizing the sodium content.

Olives: Go for olives that are not packed in oil, sparingly use them as they are very high in sodium.

12.Cheese Substitutes

You should go for nutritional yeast for sprinkling purposes on pasta and even use it in recipes for adding a "cheesy" flavor to them. Special occasion's option includes:

•Miyoko's Creamery cheeses (choose the no added oil varieties

•Miyoko's Creamery cheeses (choose the no added oil varieties

They are very high in fat, so you have to use them in a moderate manner.

Chapter 3.Snacks And Desserts

1. Thai Snack Mix

Preparation time: 15 minutes

Cooking time: 90 minutes

Servings: 4

Ingredients:

5 cups mixed nuts

1 cup chopped dried pineapple

1 cup pumpkin seed

1 teaspoon onion powder

1 teaspoon garlic powder

2 teaspoons paprika

1/2 teaspoon ground black pepper

1 teaspoon of sea salt

1/4 cup coconut sugar

1/2 teaspoon red chili powder

1 tablespoon red pepper flakes

1/2 tablespoon red curry powder

2 tablespoons soy sauce

2 tablespoons coconut oil

Directions:

Switch on the slow cooker, add all the ingredients in it except for dried pineapple and red pepper flakes, stir until combined and cook for 90 minutes at high heat setting, stirring every 30 minutes.

When done, spread the nut mixture on a baking sheet lined with parchment paper and let it cool.

Then spread dried pineapple on top, sprinkle with red pepper flakes and serve.

Nutrition:

Calories: 230 Cal

Fat: 17.5 g

Carbs: 11.5 g

Protein: 6.5 g

Fiber: 2 g

2. Zucchini Fritters

Preparation time: 10 minutes

Cooking time: 6 minutes

Servings: 12

Ingredients:

1/2 cup quinoa flour

3 1/2 cups shredded zucchini

1/2 cup chopped scallions

1/3 teaspoon ground black pepper

1 teaspoon salt

2 tablespoons coconut oil

2 flax eggs

Directions:

Squeeze moisture from the zucchini by wrapping it in a cheesecloth and then transfer it to a bowl.

Add remaining ingredients, except for oil, stir until combined and then shape the mixture into twelve patties.

Take a skillet pan, place it over medium-high heat, add oil and when hot, add patties and cook for 3 minutes per side until brown.

Serve the patties with favorite vegan sauce.

Nutrition:

Calories: 37 Cal

Fat: 1 g

Carbs: 4 g

Protein: 2 g

Fiber: 1 g

3. Zucchini Chips

Preparation time: 10 minutes

Cooking time: 120 minutes

Servings: 4

Ingredients:

1 large zucchini, thinly sliced

1 teaspoon salt

2 tablespoons olive oil

Directions:

Pat dry zucchini slices and then spread them in an even layer on a baking sheet lined with parchment sheet.

Whisk together salt and oil, brush this mixture over zucchini slices on both sides and then bake for 2 hours or more until brown and crispy.

When done, let the chips cool for 10 minutes and then serve straight away.

Nutrition:

Calories: 54 Cal

Fat: 5 g

Carbs: 1 g

Protein: 0 g

Fiber: 0.3 g

4. Rosemary Beet Chips

Preparation time: 10 minutes

Cooking time: 20 minutes

Servings: 3

Ingredients:

3 large beets, scrubbed, thinly sliced

1/8 teaspoon ground black pepper

¼ teaspoon of sea salt

3 sprigs of rosemary, leaves chopped

4 tablespoons olive oil

Directions:

Spread beet slices in a single layer between two large baking sheets, brush the slices with oil, then season with spices and rosemary, toss until well coated, and bake for 20 minutes at 375 degrees F until crispy, turning halfway.

When done, let the chips cool for 10 minutes and then serve.

Nutrition:

Calories: 79 Cal

Fat: 4.7 g

Carbs: 8.6 g

Protein: 1.5 g

Fiber: 2.5 g

5. Quinoa Broccoli Tots

Preparation time: 10 minutes

Cooking time: 20 minutes

Servings: 16

Ingredients:

2 tablespoons quinoa flour

2 cups steamed and chopped broccoli florets

1/2 cup nutritional yeast

1 teaspoon garlic powder

1 teaspoon miso paste

2 flax eggs

2 tablespoons hummus

Directions:

Place all the ingredients in a bowl, stir until well combined, and then shape the mixture into sixteen small balls.

Arrange the balls on a baking sheet lined with parchment paper, spray with oil and bake at 400 degrees F for 20 minutes until brown, turning halfway.

When done, let the tots cool for 10 minutes and then serve straight away.

Nutrition:

Calories: 19 Cal

Fat: 0 g

Carbs: 2 g

Protein: 1 g

Fiber: 0.5 g

6. Spicy Roasted Chickpeas

Preparation time: 10 minutes

Cooking time: 20 minutes

Servings: 6

Ingredients:

30 ounces cooked chickpeas

½ teaspoon salt

2 teaspoons mustard powder

½ teaspoon cayenne pepper

2 tablespoons olive oil

Directions:

Place all the ingredients in a bowl and stir until well coated and then spread the chickpeas in an even layer on a baking sheet greased with oil.

Bake the chickpeas for 20 minutes at 400 degrees F until golden brown and crispy and then serve straight away.

Nutrition:

Calories: 187.1 Cal

Fat: 7.4 g

Carbs: 24.2 g

Protein: 7.3 g

Fiber: 6.3 g

7. Nacho Kale Chips

Preparation time: 10 minutes

Cooking time: 14 hours

Servings: 10

Ingredients:

2 bunches of curly kale

2 cups cashews, soaked, drained

1/2 cup chopped red bell pepper

1 teaspoon garlic powder

1 teaspoon salt

2 tablespoons red chili powder

1/2 teaspoon smoked paprika

1/2 cup nutritional yeast

1 teaspoon cayenne

3 tablespoons lemon juice

3/4 cup water

Directions:

Place all the ingredients except for kale in a food processor and pulse for 2 minutes until smooth.

Place kale in a large bowl, pour in the blended mixture, mix until coated, and dehydrate for 14 hours at 120 degrees F until crispy.

If dehydrator is not available, spread kale between two baking sheets and bake for 90 minutes at 225 degrees F until crispy, flipping halfway.

When done, let chips cool for 15 minutes and then serve.

Nutrition:

Calories: 191 Cal

Fat: 12 g

Carbs: 16 g

Protein: 9 g

Fiber: 2 g

8. Red Salsa

Preparation time: 10 minutes

Cooking time: 0 minute

Servings: 8

Ingredients:

30 ounces diced fire-roasted tomatoes

4 tablespoons diced green chilies

1 medium jalapeño pepper, deseeded

1/2 cup chopped green onion

1 cup chopped cilantro

1 teaspoon minced garlic

½ teaspoon of sea salt

1 teaspoon ground cumin

¼ teaspoon stevia

3 tablespoons lime juice

Directions:

Place all the ingredients in a food processor and process for 2 minutes until smooth.

Tip the salsa in a bowl, taste to adjust seasoning and then serve.

Nutrition:

Calories: 71 Cal

Fat: 0.2 g

Carbs: 19 g

Protein: 2 g

Fiber: 4.1 g

9. Tomato Hummus

Preparation time: 5 minutes

Cooking time: 0 minute

Servings: 4

Ingredients:

1/4 cup sun-dried tomatoes, without oil

1 ½ cups cooked chickpeas

1 teaspoon minced garlic

1/2 teaspoon salt

2 tablespoons sesame oil

1 tablespoon lemon juice

1 tablespoon olive oil

1/4 cup of water

Directions:

Place all the ingredients in a food processor and process for 2 minutes until smooth.

Tip the hummus in a bowl, drizzle with more oil, and then serve straight away.

Nutrition:

Calories: 122.7 Cal

Fat: 4.1 g

Carbs: 17.8 g

Protein: 5.1 g

Fiber: 3.5 g

10. Marinated Mushrooms

Preparation time: 10 minutes

Cooking time: 7 minutes

Servings: 6

Ingredients:

12 ounces small button mushrooms

1 teaspoon minced garlic

1/4 teaspoon dried thyme

1/2 teaspoon sea salt

1/2 teaspoon dried basil

1/2 teaspoon red pepper flakes

1/4 teaspoon dried oregano

1/2 teaspoon maple syrup

1/4 cup apple cider vinegar

1/4 cup and 1 teaspoon olive oil

2 tablespoons chopped parsley

Directions:

Take a skillet pan, place it over medium-high heat, add 1 teaspoon oil and when hot, add mushrooms and cook for 5 minutes until golden brown.

Meanwhile, prepare the marinade and for this, place remaining ingredients in a bowl and whisk until combined.

When mushrooms have cooked, transfer them into the bowl of marinade and toss until well coated.

Serve straight away

Nutrition:

Calories: 103 Cal

Fat: 9 g

Carbs: 2 g

Protein: 1 g

Fiber: 1 g

11. Hummus Quesadillas

Preparation time: 5 minutes

Cooking time: 15 minutes

Servings: 1

Ingredients:

1 tortilla, whole wheat

1/4 cup diced roasted red peppers

1 cup baby spinach

1/3 teaspoon minced garlic

¼ teaspoon salt

¼ teaspoon ground black pepper

1/4 teaspoon olive oil

1/4 cup hummus

Oil as needed

Directions:

Place a large pan over medium heat, add oil and when hot, add red peppers and garlic, season with salt and black pepper and cook for 3 minutes until sauté.

Then stir in spinach, cook for 1 minute, remove the pan from heat and transfer the mixture in a bowl.

Prepare quesadilla and for this, spread hummus on one-half of the tortilla, then spread spinach mixture on it, cover the filling with the other half of the tortilla and cook in a pan for 3 minutes per side until browned.

When done, cut the quesadilla into wedges and serve.

Nutrition:

Calories: 187 Cal

Fat: 9 g

Carbs: 16.3 g

Protein: 10.4 g

Fiber: 0 g

12. Nacho Cheese Sauce

Preparation time: 5 minutes

Cooking time: 10 minutes

Servings: 4

Ingredients:

3 tablespoons flour

1/4 teaspoon garlic salt

1/4 teaspoon salt

1/2 teaspoon cumin

1/4 teaspoon paprika

1 teaspoon red chili powder

1/8 teaspoon cayenne powder

1 cup vegan cashew yogurt

1 1/4 cups vegetable broth

Directions:

Take a small saucepan, place it over medium heat, pour in vegetable broth, and bring it to a boil.

Then whisk together flour and yogurt, add to the boiling broth, stir in all the spices, switch heat to medium-low level and cook for 5 minutes until thickened.

Serve straight away.

Nutrition:

Calories: 282 Cal

Fat: 1 g

Carbs: 63 g

Protein: 3 g

Fiber: 12 g

13.   Avocado Tomato Bruschetta

Preparation time: 10 minutes

Cooking time: 0 minute

Servings: 4

Ingredients:

3 slices of whole-grain bread

6 chopped cherry tomatoes

½ of sliced avocado

½ teaspoon minced garlic

½ teaspoon ground black pepper

2 tablespoons chopped basil

½ teaspoon of sea salt

1 teaspoon balsamic vinegar

Directions:

Place tomatoes in a bowl, and then stir in vinegar until mixed.

Top bread slices with avocado slices, then top evenly with tomato mixture, garlic and basil, and season with salt and black pepper.

Serve straight away

Nutrition:

Calories: 131 Cal

Fat: 7.3 g

Carbs: 15 g

Protein: 2.8 g

Fiber: 3.2 g

14.   Cinnamon Bananas

Preparation time: 5 minutes

Cooking time: 8 minutes

Servings: 2

Ingredients:

2 bananas, peeled, sliced

1 teaspoon cinnamon

2 tablespoons granulated Splenda

1/4 teaspoon nutmeg

Directions:

Prepare the cinnamon mixture and for this, place all the ingredients in a bowl, except for banana, and stir until mixed.

Take a large skillet pan, place it over medium heat, spray with oil, add banana slices and sprinkle with half of the prepared cinnamon mixture.

Cook for 3 minutes, then sprinkle with remaining prepared cinnamon mixture and continue cooking for 3 minutes until tender and hot.

Serve straight away.

Nutrition:

Calories: 155 Cal

Fat: 2 g

Carbs: 39 g

Protein: 1 g

Fiber: 3 g

15.   Salted Almonds

Preparation time: 5 minutes

Cooking time: 20 minutes

Servings: 4

Ingredients:

2 cups almonds

4 tablespoons salt

1 cup boiling water

Directions:

Stir the salt into the boiling water in a pan, then add almonds in it and let them soak for 20 minutes.

Then drain the almonds, spread them in an even layer on a baking sheet lined with baking paper and sprinkle with salt.

Roast the almonds for 20 minutes at 300 degrees F, then cool them for 10 minutes and serve.

Nutrition:

Calories: 170 Cal

Fat: 16 g

Carbs: 5 g

Protein: 6 g

Fiber: 3 g

16.   Pumpkin Cake Pops

Preparation time: 10 minutes

Cooking time: 10 minutes

Servings: 4

Ingredients:

1 cup coconut flour

¼ teaspoon cinnamon

1/4 cup coconut sugar

1/4 cup chocolate chips, unsweetened

3/4 cup pumpkin puree

Directions:

Place all the ingredients in a bowl, except for chocolate chips, stir until incorporated, and then fold in chocolate chips until combined.

Shape the mixture into small balls, then place them on a cookie sheet greased with oil and bake for 10 minutes at 350 degrees F until done.

Let the balls cool completely and then serve.

Nutrition:

Calories: 82.5 Cal

Fat: 3.4 g

Carbs: 12.3 g

Protein: 0.7 g

Fiber: 0.05 g

17. Honey-Almond Popcorn

Preparation time: 5 minutes

Cooking time: 10 minutes

Servings: 4

Ingredients:

1/2 cup popcorn kernels

2 tablespoons honey

1/2 teaspoon sea salt

2 tablespoons coconut sugar

1 cup roasted almonds

1/4 cup walnut oil

Directions:

Take a pot, place it over medium-low heat, add oil and when it melts, add four kernels and wait until they sizzle.

Then add remaining kernel, toss until coated, sprinkle with sugar, drizzle with honey, shut the pot with the lid, and shake the kernels until popped completely, adding almonds halfway.

Once all the kernels have popped, season them with salt and serve straight away.

Nutrition:

Calories: 120 Cal

Fat: 4.5 g

Carbs: 19 g

Protein: 1 g

Fiber: 1 g

18.   Turmeric Snack Bites

Preparation time: 35 minutes

Cooking time: 0 minute

Servings: 10

Ingredients:

1 cup Medjool dates, pitted, chopped

1/2 cup walnuts

1 teaspoon ground turmeric

1 tablespoon cocoa powder, unsweetened

1/2 teaspoon ground cinnamon

1/2 cup shredded coconut, unsweetened

Directions:

Place all the ingredients in a food processor and pulse for 2 minutes until a smooth mixture comes together.

Tip the mixture in a bowl and then shape it into ten small balls, 1 tablespoon of the mixture per ball and then refrigerate for 30 minutes.

Serve straight away.

Nutrition:

Calories: 109 Cal

Fat: 2 g

Carbs: 13 g

Protein: 1 g

Fiber: 0 g

19. Watermelon Pizza

Preparation time: 10 minutes

Cooking time: 0 minute

Servings: 10

Ingredients:

1/2 cup strawberries, halved

1/2 cup blueberries

1 watermelon

1/2 cup raspberries

1 cup of coconut yogurt

1/2 cup pomegranate seeds

1/2 cup cherries

Maple syrup as needed

Directions:

Cut watermelon into 3-inch thick slices, then spread yogurt on one side, leaving some space in the edges and then top evenly with fruits and drizzle with maple syrup.

Cut the watermelon into wedges and then serve.

Nutrition:

Calories: 150 Cal

Fat: 4 g

Carbs: 21 g

Protein: 10 g

Fiber: 2 g

20. Rosemary Popcorn

Preparation time: 10 minutes

Cooking time: 10 minutes

Servings: 4

Ingredients:

1/2 cup popcorn kernels

1/2 teaspoon sea salt

1 tablespoon and 1/2 teaspoon minced rosemary

3 tablespoons unsalted vegan butter

1/4 cup olive oil

1/3 teaspoon ground black pepper

Directions:

Take a pot, place it over medium-low heat, add oil and when it melts, add four kernels and wait until they sizzle.

Then add remaining kernel, toss until coated, add 1 tablespoon minced rosemary, shut the pot with the lid, and shake the kernels until popped completely.

Once all the kernels have popped, transfer them in a bowl, cook remaining rosemary into melted butter, then drizzle this mixture over popcorn and toss until well coated.

Season popcorn with salt and black pepper, toss until mixed and serve.

Nutrition:

Calories: 160 Cal

Fat: 6 g

Carbs: 28 g

Protein: 3 g

Fiber: 4 g

21.   Queso Dip

Preparation time: 5 minutes

Cooking time: 0 minute

Servings: 6

Ingredients:

1 cup cashews

½ teaspoon minced garlic

1/2 teaspoon salt

1/2 teaspoon ground cumin

1 teaspoon red chili powder

2 tablespoons nutritional yeast

1 tablespoon harissa

1 cup hot water

Directions:

Place all the ingredients in a food processor and pulse for 2 minutes until smooth and well combined.

Tip the dip in a bowl, taste to adjust seasoning and then serve.

Nutrition:

Calories: 133 Cal

Fat: 9 g

Carbs: 8 g

Protein: 5 g

Fiber: 1 g

22. Nooch Popcorn

Preparation time: 10 minutes

Cooking time: 10 minutes

Servings: 4

Ingredients:

1/3 cup nutritional yeast

1 teaspoon of sea salt

3 tablespoons coconut oil

½ cup popcorn kernels

Directions:

Place yeast in a large bowl, stir in salt, and set aside until required.

Take a medium saucepan, place it over medium-high heat, add oil and when it melts, add four kernels and wait until they sizzle.

Then add remaining kernel, toss until coated, shut the pan with the lid, and shake the kernels until popped completely.

When done, transfer popcorns tot eh yeast mixture, shut with lid and shape well until coated.

Serve straight away

Nutrition:

Calories: 160 Cal

Fat: 6 g

Carbs: 28 g

Protein: 3 g

Fiber: 4 g

23.   Masala Popcorn

Preparation time: 5 minutes

Cooking time: 15 minutes

Servings: 4

Ingredients:

3 cups popped popcorn

2 hot chili peppers, sliced

1 teaspoon ground cumin

6 curry leaves

1 teaspoon ground coriander

1/3 teaspoon salt

1/8 teaspoon chaat masala

1/4 teaspoon turmeric powder

¼ teaspoon red pepper flakes

1/4 teaspoon garam masala

1/3 cup olive oil

Directions:

Take a large pot, place it over medium heat, add half of the oil and when hot, add chili peppers and curry leaves and cook for 3 minutes until golden.

When done, transfer curry leaves and pepper to a plate lined with paper towels and set aside until required.

Add remaining oil into the pot, add remaining ingredients except for popcorns, stir until mixed and cook for 1 minute until fragrant.

Then tip in popcorns, remove the pan from heat, stir well until coated, and then sprinkle with bay leaves and red chili.

Toss until mixed and serve straight away.

Nutrition:

Calories: 150 Cal

Fat: 9 g

Carbs: 15 g

Protein: 2 g

Fiber: 4 g

24.   Applesauce

Preparation time: 10 minutes

Cooking time: 15 minutes

Servings: 6

Ingredients:

4 pounds mixed apples, cored, ½-inch chopped

1 strip of orange peel, about 3-inch

1/2 cup coconut sugar

1/2 teaspoon salt

1 cinnamon stick, about 3-inch

2 tablespoons apple cider vinegar

Apple cider as needed for consistency of the sauce

Directions:

Take a large pot, place apples in it, then add remaining ingredients except for cider, stir until mixed and cook for 15 minutes over medium heat until apples have wilted, stirring every 10 minutes.

When done, remove the cinnamon stick and orange peel and puree the mixture by using an immersion blender until smooth and stir in apple cider until sauce reaches to desired consistency.

Serve straight away.

Nutrition:

Calories: 75 Cal

Fat: 0.2 g

Carbs: 19 g

Protein: 0.2 g

Fiber: 1.3 g

25.   Avocado Toast with Herbs and Peas

Preparation time: 10 minutes

Cooking time: 0 minute

Servings: 4

Ingredients:

½ of a medium avocado, peeled, pitted, mashed

6 slices of radish

2 tablespoons baby peas

¼ teaspoon ground black pepper

1 teaspoon chopped basil

¼ teaspoon salt

1/2 lemon, juiced

1 slice of bread, whole-grain, toasted

Directions:

Spread mashed avocado on the one side of the toast and then top with peas, pressing them into the avocado.

Layer the toast with radish slices, season with salt and black pepper, sprinkle with basil, and drizzle with lemon juice.

Serve straight away.

Nutrition:

Calories: 250 Cal

Fat: 12 g

Carbs: 22 g

Protein: 7 g

Fiber: 9 g

26. Oven-Dried Grapes

Preparation time: 5 minutes

Cooking time: 4 hours

Servings: 4

Ingredients:

3 large bunches of grapes, seedless

Olive oil as needed for greasing

Directions:

Spread grapes into two greased baking sheets and bake for 4 hours at 225 degrees F until semi-dried.

When done, let the grape cool completely and then serve.

Nutrition:

Calories: 299 Cal

Fat: 1 g

Carbs: 79 g

Protein: 3.1 g

Fiber: 3.7 g

27.   Black Bean and Corn Quesadillas

Preparation time: 15 minutes

Cooking time: 30 minutes

Servings: 4

Ingredients:

For the Black Beans and Corn:

1/2 of a medium white onion, peeled, chopped

1/2 cup cooked black beans

1/2 cup cooked corn kernels

1 teaspoon minced garlic

½ of jalapeno, deseeded, diced

1/2 teaspoon salt

1 teaspoon red chili powder

1 teaspoon cumin

1 tablespoon olive oil

For the Quesadillas:

4 large corn tortillas

4 green onions, chopped

½ cup vegan nacho cheese sauce

½ cup chopped cilantro

1 large tomato, diced

Salsa as needed for dipping

Directions:

Prepare beans and for this, take a frying pan, place it over medium-high heat, add oil and when hot, add onion, jalapeno, and garlic and cook for 3 minutes.

Then add remaining ingredients, stir until mixed and cook for 2 minutes until hot.

Take a large skillet pan, place over medium heat, place the tortilla in it and cook for 1 minute until toasted and then flip it.

Spread some of the cheese sauce on one half of the top, spread with beans mixture, top with cilantro, onion, and tomato and then fold the filling with the other side of the tortilla.

Pat down the tortilla, cook it for 2 minutes, then carefully flip it, continue cooking for 2 minutes until hot, and then slide to a plate.

Cook remaining quesadilla in the same manner, then cut them into wedges and serve.

Nutrition:

Calories: 251 Cal

Fat: 9.5 g

Carbs: 30.6 g

Protein: 15.6 g

Fiber: 12.1 g

28. Mint Chocolate Cheesecake

Preparation Time: 10minutes

Cooking Time: 5minutes, 3.5 hours refrigeration

Servings: 4

Ingredients:

For the crust:

1 cup raw almonds

½ cup salted butter, melted

2 tbsp swerve sugar

For the cake:

4 tbsp unsalted butter, melted

2 vegan sheets

2 tbsp lime juice

2/3 cup unsweetened dark chocolate, chopped + extra for garnishing

1 ½ cups cashew cream

½ cup swerve sugar

1 cup Greek sugar free coconut yogurt

1 tbsp mint extract

Directions:

For the crust:

Preheat the oven to 350 F.

In a blender, process the almonds until finely ground. Add the butter and sweetener, and mix until combined.

Press the crust mixture into the bottom of the cake pan until firm.

Bake for 5 minutes. Place in the fridge to chill afterward.

For the cake:

In a small pot, combine the vegan with the lime juice, and a tablespoon of water. Allow sitting for 5 minutes and then, place the pot over medium heat to dissolve the vegan. Set aside.

Pour the dark chocolate in a bowl and melt in the microwave for 1 minute, stirring at every 10 seconds interval. Set aside.

In another, beat the cashew cream and swerve sugar using an electric mixer until smooth. Stir in the sugar free coconut yogurt and vegan until evenly combined. After, fold in the melted dark chocolate and then the mint extract.

Remove the pan from the fridge and pour the cream mixture on top. Tap the side gently to release any trapped air bubbles and transfer to the fridge to chip for 3 hours or more.

When ready, remove and release the pan's locker, garnish the top if the cake with more dark chocolate, and slice.

Serve immediately.

Nutrition

Calories: 687, Total Fat:54.4g, Saturated Fat:27.4g, Total Carbs: 9g, Dietary Fiber:2g, Sugar:4 g, Protein:38 g, Sodium: 883mg

29.   Blueberry Smoothie

Preparation Time: 5

Servings: 4

Ingredients:

2 cups fresh blueberries

1 cup almond milk

½ cup heavy cream

Sugar-free maple syrup to taste

2 tbsp sesame seeds

Chopped pistachios for topping

1 tbsp chopped mint leaves

Directions:

Combine the blueberries, milk, heavy cream, and syrup in a blender.

Process until smooth and pour into serving glasses.

Top with the sesame seeds, pistachios, and mint leaves.

Serve immediately.

Nutrition

Calories:260 , Total Fat:24.7g, Saturated Fat:14.3g, Total Carbs: 4g, Dietary Fiber:0g, Sugar: 6g, Protein: 2g, Sodium:215 mg

30.   Zucchini Cake Slices

Preparation Time: 10munites

Cooking Time: 20minutes

Servings: 4

Ingredients:

1 cup butter, softened + extra for greasing

1 cup erythritol

4 eggs

2/3 cup coconut flour

2 tsp baking powder

2/3 cup ground almonds

1 lemon, zested and juiced

1 cup finely grated zucchini

1 cup crème fraiche, for serving

1 tbsp chopped walnuts

Directions:

Preheat the oven to 375 F, grease a springform pan with cooking spray, and line with parchment paper.

In a bowl, beat the butter and erythritol until creamy and pale. Add the eggs one after another while whisking. Sift the coconut flour and baking powder into the mixture and stir along with the ground almonds, lemon zest, juice, and zucchini.

Spoon the mixture into the springform pan and bake in the oven for 40 minutes or until risen and a toothpick inserted into the cake comes out clean.

Remove the cake from the oven when ready; allow cooling in the pan for 10 minutes, and transfer to a wire rack.

Spread the crème fraiche on top of the cake and sprinkle with the walnuts. Slice and serve.

Nutrition

Calories:262 , Total Fat:27.7g, Saturated Fat:13.3g, Total Carbs: 4g, Dietary Fiber:0g, Sugar: 6g, Protein: 2g, Sodium:215 mg

31. Mixed Berry Pie

Preparation Time: 10minutes

Cooking Time: 20minutes, 2hour refrigeration

Servings: 4

Ingredients:

For the piecrust:

¼ cup almond flour + extra for dusting

3 tbsp coconut flour

½ tsp salt

¼ cup butter, cold and crumbled

3 tbsp erythritol

1 ½ tsp vanilla extract

4 whole eggs

For the filling:

2 ¼ cup strawberries and blackberries

1 cup erythritol + extra for sprinkling

1 vanilla pod, bean paste extracted

1 egg, beaten

Directions:

Preheat the oven to 350 F and grease a pie pan with cooking spray

In a large bowl, mix the almond flour, coconut flour, and salt.

Add the butter and mix with an electric hand mixer until crumbly. Add the erythritol and vanilla extract until mixed in. Then, pour in the 4 eggs one after another while mixing until formed into a ball.

Flatten the dough a clean flat surface, cover in plastic wrap, and refrigerate for 1 hour.

After, lightly dust a clean flat surface with almond flour, unwrap the dough, and roll out the dough into a large rectangle, ½ - inch thickness and fit into a pie pan.

Pour some baking beans onto the pastry and bake in the oven until golden. Remove after, pour pout the baking beans, and allow cooling.

In a bowl, mix the berries, erythritol, and vanilla bean paste. Spoon the mixture into the pie, level with a spoon, and use the pastry strips to create a lattice top over the berries. Brush with the beaten egg, sprinkle with more erythritol, and bake for 30 minutes or until the fruit is bubbling and the pie golden brown.

Remove from the oven, allow cooling, slice, and serve with whipped cream

Nutrition

Calories:238 , Total Fat:26.3g, Saturated Fat:14.9g, Total Carbs: 1g, Dietary Fiber:0g, Sugar:0 g, Protein:1 g, Sodium:183 mg

32.   Blackberry Lemon Tarte Tatin

Preparation Time: 10minutes

Cooking Time: 40minutes

Servings: 4

Ingredients:

For the piecrust:

¼ cup almond flour + extra for dusting

3 tbsp coconut flour

½ tsp salt

¼ cup butter, cold and crumbled

3 tbsp erythritol

1 ½ tsp vanilla extract

4 whole eggs

For the filling:

4 tbsp melted butter

3 tsp swerve brown sugar

1 cup fresh blackberries

1 tsp vanilla extract

1 lemon, juiced

1 cup ricotta cheese

3 to 4 fresh basil leaves to garnish

1 egg, lightly beaten

Directions:

For the piecrust:

Preheat the oven to 350 F and grease a pie pan with cooking spray

In a large bowl, mix the almond flour, coconut flour, and salt.

Add the butter and mix with an electric hand mixer until crumbly. Add the erythritol and vanilla extract until mixed in. Then, pour in the 4 eggs one after another while mixing until formed into a ball.

Flatten the dough a clean flat surface, cover in plastic wrap, and refrigerate for 1 hour.

After, lightly dust a clean flat surface with almond flour, unwrap the dough, and roll out the dough into a 1-inch diameter circle.

For the filling:

In a 10-inch shallow baking pan, mix the butter, swerve brown sugar, blackberries, vanilla extract, and lemon juice. Arrange the blackberries uniformly across the pan.

Lay the pastry over the fruit filling and tuck the sides into the pan. Brush with the beaten egg and bake in the oven for 35 to 40 minutes or until the golden and puffed up.

Remove, allow cooling for 5 minutes, and then run a knife around the pan to losing the pastry. Turn the pie over onto a plate, crumble the ricotta cheese on top, and garnish with the basil leaves.

Nutrition

Calories: 15, Total Fat:1.3g, Saturated Fat:0.1g, Total Carbs: 1g, Dietary Fiber:0g, Sugar:1 g, Protein: 1g, Sodium:8 mg

33.   Lemon Sponge Cake with Cream

Preparation Time: 10minutes

Cooking Time: 30minutes

Servings: 4

Ingredients:

For the lemon puree:

4 large lemons

¼ cup sugar-free maple syrup

¼ tsp salt

For the cake:

½ cup unsalted butter, softened

½ cup erythritol

1 tsp vanilla extract

½ cup almond flour, sifted

3 large eggs, lightly beaten

½ cup heavy cream

1 tbsp swerve confectioner's sugar, for dusting

Directions:

For the lemon puree:

Peel and juice the lemon. Strain or remove any white strains from the peel and transfer both peels and juice to a small saucepan. Add the erythritol and salt and simmer over low heat for 30 minutes.

Pour the mixture into a blender and process until smooth. Pour into a jar and set aside.

For the cake:

Preheat the oven to 350 F, grease a two (2 x 8 inchspringform pans with cooking spray, and line with parchment paper.

In a large mixing bowl, cream the butter, erythritol, and vanilla extract with an electric whisk until light and fluffy. Pour in the eggs gradually while beating until fully mixed. Carefully fold in the almond flour and share the mixture into the cake pans.

Bake in the oven for 25 to 30 minutes or until springy when touched and a toothpick inserted comes out clean.

Remove and allow cooling in the pans for 5 minutes before turning out onto a wire rack.

In a bowl, whip the double cream until a soft peak forms. Spoon onto the bottom sides of the cake and spread the lemon puree on top. Sandwich both cakes and sift the confectioner's sugar on top.

Slice and serve.

Nutrition

Calories:304 , Total Fat:29g, Saturated Fat:23.5g, Total Carbs: 8g, Dietary Fiber:3g, Sugar:1 g, Protein:8 g, Sodium: 8mg

34.   Dark Chocolate Fudge

Preparation Time: 10minutes

Cooking Time: 20minutes

Servings: 4

Ingredients:

4 large eggs

1 cup swerve sugar

1 cup unsweetened dark chocolate, melted

½ cup melted butter

1/3 cup coconut flour

Directions:

Preheat the oven to 350 F and line a rectangular baking tray with parchment paper.

In a large mixing bowl, cream the eggs with swerve sugar until smooth. Add the melted chocolate, butter, and whisk until evenly combined. Carefully fold in the coconut flour to incorporate and pour the mixture into the baking tray.

Bake in the oven for 20 minutes or until a toothpick inserted comes out clean.

Remove from the oven and allow cooling in the tray. After, cut into squares and serve.

Nutrition

Calories:412 , Total Fat:43g, Saturated Fat:37g, Total Carbs: 9g, Dietary Fiber:3g, Sugar:0 g, Protein: 5g, Sodium:12 mg

35. Creamy Avocado Drink

Preparation Time: 5minutes

Servings: 4

Ingredients:

4 large ripe avocados, halved and pitted

4 tbsp swerve sugar

¼ cup cold almond milk

1 tsp vanilla extract

1 tbsp cold heavy cream

Directions:

In a blender, add the avocado pulp, swerve sugar, almond milk, vanilla extract, and heavy cream. Process until smooth.

Pour the mixture into 2 tall serving glasses, garnish with strawberries, and serve immediately.

Nutrition

Calories: 193, Total Fat:20.1g, Saturated Fat12,5g, Total Carbs: 3g, Dietary Fiber:0g, Sugar:2 g, Protein:1g, Sodium:100 mg

36.   Walnut Chocolate Squares

Preparation Time: 5minutes

Cooking Time: 3minutes

Servings: 6

Ingredients:

3½ oz. dairy-free dark chocolate, unsweetened

4 tbsp butter

1 pinch salt

¼ cup walnut butter

½ tsp vanilla extract

¼ cup chopped walnuts to garnish

Directions:

Pour the chocolate and butter in a safe microwave bowl and melt in the microwave for about 1 to 2 minutes.

Remove the bowl from the microwave and mix in the salt, walnut butter, and vanilla extract.

Grease a small baking sheet with cooking spray and line with parchment paper. Pour in the batter and use a spatula to spread out into a 4 x 6-inch rectangle.

Top with the chopped walnuts and chill in the refrigerator.

Once set, cut into 1 x 1-inch squares.

Serve while firming.

Nutrition

Calories:132 , Total Fat:11.5g, Saturated Fat:4.3g, Total Carbs: 7g, Dietary Fiber:4g, Sugar:2 g, Protein: 1g, Sodium:10 mg

37. Cacao Nut Bites

Preparation Time: 2 minutes

Cooking Time: 2 minutes

Servings 4

Ingredients:

3½ oz. dairy-free dark chocolate

½ cup mixed nuts (hazelnuts, walnuts, pecans

2 tbsp roasted unsweetened coconut chips

1 tbsp sunflower seeds

Sea salt

Directions:

Pour the chocolate into a safe microwave bowl and melt in the microwave for 1 to 2 minutes.

Into 10 small cupcake liners (2-inches in diameters), share the chocolate.

Drop in the nuts, coconut chips, sunflower seeds and sprinkle with some salt.

Chill in the refrigerator until firm.

Serve immediately.

Nutrition

Calories:130 , Total Fat:12.4g, Saturated Fat:4.3g, Total Carbs: 6g, Dietary Fiber:4g, Sugar:0 g, Protein: 1g, Sodium: 5mg

38.   Cinnamon Tofu Pudding

Preparation Time: 17minutes

Servings: 6

Ingredients:

1¼ cups coconut cream

1 tsp vanilla extract

1 tsp cinnamon powder

1 cup tofu cheese

2 oz. fresh strawberries

Directions:

Pour the coconut cream into a bowl and whisk until a soft peak forms. Mix in the vanilla and cinnamon.

Lightly fold in the tofu cheese and refrigerate for 10 to 15 minutes to set.

Spoon into serving glasses, top with the strawberries and serve immediately.

Nutrition

Calories:114 , Total Fat:11.8g, Saturated Fat:7.4g, Total Carbs: 1g, Dietary Fiber:1g, Sugar: 1g, Protein:1 g, Sodium: 39mg

39. Raspberries Turmeric Panna Cotta

Preparation Time: 3minutes, 2hours refrigeration

Cooking Time: 4minutes

Servings: 6

Ingredients:

½ tbsp unflavored powdered vegan + ½ tsp water

2 cups coconut cream

¼ tsp vanilla extract

1 pinch turmeric powder

1 tbsp erythritol

1 tbsp chopped toasted pecans

12 fresh raspberries

Directions

Mix the vegan and water and allow sitting to dissolve.

Pour the coconut cream, vanilla extract, turmeric, and erythritol into a saucepan and bring to a boil over medium heat, then, simmer for 2 minutes. Turn the heat off.

Pour the mixture into 6 glasses, cover with a plastic wrap, and refrigerate for 2 hours or more.

Remove, top with the pecans and raspberries, and serve immediately.

Nutrition

Calories:830 , Total Fat:86.9g, Saturated Fat:44.7g, Total Carbs: 12g, Dietary Fiber:3g, Sugar: 7g, Protein: 6g, Sodium: 395mg

40.   White Chocolate Fudge

Preparation Time: 5minutes

Cooking Time: 15 minutes, 4 hours refrigeration

Servings: 6

Ingredients:

2 cups coconut cream

1 tsp vanilla extract

3 oz. butter

3 oz. unsweetened white chocolate

Swerve sugar for sprinkling

Directions:

Pour the coconut cream and vanilla into a saucepan and bring to a boil over medium heat, then simmer until reduced by half, about 15 minutes.

Stir in the butter until the batter is smooth; turn the heat off.

Chop the white chocolate into small bits and stir into the cream until melted.

Pour the mixture into a 7 x 7 baking sheet and chill in the fridge for 3 to 4 hours.

After, cut into squares, sprinkle with a little swerve sugar, and serve.

Nutrition

Calories:297 , Total Fat:31.3g, Saturated Fat:25g, Total Carbs: 5g, Dietary Fiber:1g, Sugar:1 g, Protein:3g, Sodium:14 mg

41. Cheesecake with Blueberries

Preparation Time: 4minutes

Cooking Time: 1hour, 28minutes, overnight refrigeration

Servings: 6

Ingredients:

For the piecrust:

2 oz. butter

1¼ cups almond flour

2 tbsp Swerve sugar

½ tsp vanilla extract

For the filling:

3 tbsp flax seed powder + 9 tbsp water

2 cups dairy-free cashew cream

½ cup coconut cream

1 tbsp Swerve sugar

1 tsp lemon zest

½ tsp vanilla extract

2 oz. fresh blueberries

Directions:

Preheat the oven to 350 F and grease a 9-inch springform pan with cooking spray. Line with parchment paper.

To make the crust, melt the butter in a skillet over low heat until nutty in flavor. Turn the heat off and stir in the almond flour, swerve sugar, and vanilla until a dough forms.

Press the mixture into the springform pan and bake in the oven until the crust is lightly golden, about 8 minutes.

For the filling, mix the flax seed powder with water and allow sitting for 5 minutes to thicken.

In a bowl, evenly combine the cashew cream, coconut cream, swerve sugar, lemon zest, vanilla extract, and flax egg.

Remove the crust from the oven and pour the mixture on top. Use a spatula to layer evenly.

Bake the cake for 15 minutes at 400 F.

Then, reduce the heat 230 F and bake further for 45 to 60 minutes.

Remove to cool completely. Refrigerate overnight and scatter the blueberries on top.

Unlock, lift the pan and slice the cake into wedges. Serve immediately.

Nutrition

Calories:598 , Total Fat:56g, Saturated Fat:18.8g, Total Carbs: 12g, Dietary Fiber:3g, Sugar:5 g, Protein:15 g, Sodium:762 mg

42. Lime Ice Cream

Preparation Time: 10minutes

Servings 4

Ingredients:

2 large avocados, pitted

Juice and zest of 3 limes

1/3 cup erythritol

1¾ cups coconut cream

¼ tsp vanilla extract

Directions:

In a blender, combine the avocado pulp, lime juice and zest, erythritol, coconut cream, and vanilla extract. Process until the mixture is smooth.

Pour the mixture into your ice cream maker and freeze based on the manufacturer's instructions.

When ready, remove and scoop the ice cream into bowls. Serve immediately.

Nutrition

Calories:129 , Total Fat:8.2g, Saturated Fat:5.2g, Total Carbs: 7g, Dietary Fiber:1g, Sugar: 4g, Protein:7 g, Sodium: 52mg

43.   Berry Coconut Yogurt Ice Pops

Preparation Time: 2 minutes, 8 hours refrigeration

Servings: 6

Ingredients:

2/3 cup avocado, halved and pitted

2/3 cup frozen strawberries & blueberries, thawed

1 cup dairy-free sugar free coconut yogurt

½ cup coconut cream

1 tsp vanilla extract

Directions:

Pour the avocado pulp, berries, dairy-free sugar free coconut yogurt, coconut cream, and vanilla extract. Process until smooth.

Pour into ice pop sleeves and freeze for 8 or more hours.

Enjoy the ice pops when ready.

Nutrition

Calories:240 , Total Fat:22.5g, Saturated Fat:13.8g, Total Carbs: 9g, Dietary Fiber:2g, Sugar: 6g, Protein:3 g, Sodium: 37mg

44.   Berry Hazelnut Trifle

Preparation Time: 5minutes

Servings: 4

Ingredients:

1 ½ ripe avocado

¾ cup coconut cream

Zest and juice of ½ a lemon

1 tbsp vanilla extract

3 oz. fresh strawberries

2 oz. toasted hazelnuts

Directions:

In a bowl, add the avocado pulp, coconut cream, lemon zest and juice, and half of the vanilla extract. Mix the Ingredients with an immersion blender.

Put the strawberries and remaining vanilla in another bowl and use a fork to mash the fruits.

In a tall glass, alternate layering the cream and strawberry mixtures.

Drop a few hazelnuts on each and serve the dessert immediately.

Nutrition

Calories:321 , Total Fat:31.4g, Saturated Fat:19.2g, Total Carbs: 10g, Dietary Fiber:5g, Sugar:4 g, Protein: 2g, Sodium: 298mg

45.   Avocado Truffles

Preparation Time: 4minutes

Cooking Time: 1minutes

Servings: 6

Ingredients:

1 ripe avocado, pitted

½ tsp vanilla extract

½ tsp lemon zest

1 pinch salt

5 oz. dairy-free dark chocolate, unsweetened

1 tbsp coconut oil

1 tbsp unsweetened cocoa powder

Directions:

Scoop the pulp of the avocado into a bowl and mix with the vanilla using an immersion blender. Stir in the lemon zest and a pinch of salt.

Pour the chocolate and coconut oil into a safe microwave bowl and melt in the microwave for 1 minute.

Add to the avocado mixture and stir. Allow cooling to firm up a bit.

Oil your hands with a little oil and form balls out of the mix.

Roll each ball in the cocoa powder and serve immediately.

Nutrition

Calories: 503, Total Fat:50g, Saturated Fat:30.9g, Total Carbs: 13g, Dietary Fiber:4g, Sugar: 7g, Protein:4 g, Sodium: 49mg

46.   Mint Ice Cream

Preparation Time: 10minutes, refrigeration time

Servings: 4

Ingredients:

2 avocados, pitted

1¼ cups coconut cream

½ tsp vanilla extract

2 tbsp erythritol

2 tsp chopped mint leaves

Directions:

Into a blender, spoon the avocado pulps, pour in the coconut cream, vanilla extract, erythritol, and mint leaves.

Process until smooth.

Pour the mixture into your ice cream maker and freeze according to the manufacturer's instructions.

When ready, remove and scoop the ice cream into bowls. Serve immediately.

Nutrition

Calories:373 , Total Fat:39.8 g, Saturated Fat: 24.7g, Total Carbs: 2 g, Dietary Fiber:0g, Sugar:2 g, Protein: 2g, Sodium:147 mg

47. Cardamom Coconut Fat Bombs

Preparation Time: 5minutes

Cooking Time: 2minutes

Servings: 6

Ingredients:

½ cup unsweetened grated coconut

3 oz. unsalted butter, room temperature

¼ tsp green cardamom powder

½ tsp vanilla extract

¼ tsp cinnamon powder

Directions:

Pour the grated coconut into a skillet and roast until lightly brown. Set aside to cool.

In a bowl, combine the butter, half of the coconut, cardamom, vanilla, and cinnamon.

Use your hands to form bite-size balls from the mixture and roll each in the remaining coconut.

Refrigerate the balls until ready to serve.

Nutrition

Calories:687 , Total Fat: 54.5g, Saturated Fat:27.4 g, Total Carbs: 9g, Dietary Fiber:2g, Sugar: 4g, Protein: 38g, Sodium:883 mg

48. Berries, Nuts, and Cream Bowl

Preparation Time: 10minutes

Cooking Time: 20minutes

Servings: 6

Ingredients:

For the dark chocolate cake:

5 tbsp flax seed powder + 2/3 cup water

1 cup dairy-free dark chocolate

1 cup butter

1 pinch salt

1 tsp vanilla extract

For the topping:

2 cups fresh blueberries

4 tbsp lemon juice

1 tsp vanilla extract

2 cups coconut cream

4 oz. walnuts, chopped

½ cup roasted unsweetened coconut chips

Directions:

Preheat the oven to 320 F; grease a 9-inch springform pan with cooking spray and line with parchment paper.

In a bowl, mix the flax seed powder with water and allow thickening for 5 minutes.

Then, break the chocolate and butter into a bowl and melt in the microwave for 1 to 2 minutes.

Share the flax egg into two bowls; whisk the salt into one portion and then, 1 teaspoon of vanilla into the other.

Pour the chocolate mixture into the vanilla mixture and combine well. Then, fold into the other flax egg mixture.

Pour the batter into the springform pan and bake for 15 to 20 minutes or until a knife inserted into the cake comes out clean.

When ready, slice the cake into squares and share into serving bowls. Set aside.

Pour the blueberries, lemon juice, and the remaining vanilla into a small bowl. Use a fork to break the blueberries and allow sitting for a few minutes.

Whip the coconut cream with a whisk until a soft peak forms.

To serve, spoon the cream on the cakes, top with the blueberry mixture, and sprinkle with the walnuts and coconut flakes.

Serve immediately.

Nutrition

Calories:49 , Total Fat: 45g, Saturated Fat: 29.9g, Total Carbs:12 g, Dietary Fiber:3g, Sugar: 6g, Protein: 3g, Sodium: 48mg

49. Chocolate Peppermint Mousse

Preparation Time: 10minutes, 30minutes refrigeration

Servings: 4

Ingredients:

¼ cup swerve sugar, divided

4 oz. dairy-free cashew cream, softened

3 tbsp unsweetened cocoa powder

¾ tsp peppermint extract

¼ cup warm water

½ tsp vanilla extract

1/3 cup coconut cream

Directions:

Put 2 tablespoons of swerve sugar, the cashew cream, and cocoa powder in a blender. Add the peppermint extract, warm water, and process until smooth.

In a large bowl, whip the vanilla extract, coconut cream, and the remaining swerve sugar using a whisk. Fetch out 5 to 6 tablespoons for garnishing.

Next, fold in the cocoa mixture until thoroughly combined.

Spoon the mousse into serving cups and chill in the fridge for 30 minutes.

Garnish with the reserved whipped cream and serve immediately.

Nutrition

Calories:70 , Total Fat7.4: g, Saturated Fat: 4.6g, Total Carbs: 1g, Dietary Fiber:0g, Sugar:0 g, Protein: 0g, Sodium:8 mg

50. Keto Brownies

Preparation Time: 10minutes

Cooking Time: 20minutes, 2hour refrigeration

Servings: 4

Ingredients:

2 tbsp flax seed powder + 6 tbsp water

1/4 cup unsweetened cocoa powder

1/2 cup almond flour

1/2 tsp baking powder

½ cup erythritol

10 tablespoons butter 1/2 cup + 2 tbsp

2 oz dairy-free dark chocolate

½ teaspoon vanilla extract optional

Directions:

Preheat the oven to 375 F and line a baking sheet with parchment paper. Set aside.

Mix the flax seed powder with water in a bowl and allow thickening for 5 minutes.

In a separate bowl, mix the cocoa powder, almond flour, baking powder, and erythritol until no lumps from the erythritol remain.

In another bowl, add the butter and dark chocolate and melt both in the microwave for 30 seconds to 1 minute.

Whisk the flax egg and vanilla into the chocolate mixture, then pour the mixture into the dry Ingredients. Combine evenly.

Pour the batter onto the paper-lined baking sheet and bake in the oven for 20 minutes or until a toothpick inserted into the cake comes out clean.

Remove from the oven to cool completely and refrigerate for 30 minutes to 2 hours.

When ready, slice into squares, and serve.

Nutrition

Calories: 321, Total Fat: 40.3g, Saturated Fat:18 g, Total Carbs: 19 g, Dietary Fiber:5g, Sugar:4 g, Protein:2 g, Sodium:265 mg

51. Chia Bars

Preparation time: 10 minutes

Cooking time: 20 minutes

Servings: 6

Ingredients:

1 cup coconut oil, melted

½ teaspoon baking soda

3 tablespoons chia seeds

2 tablespoons stevia

1 cup coconut cream

3 tablespoons flaxseed mixed with 4 tablespoons water

Directions:

In a bowl, combine the coconut oil with the cream, the chia seeds and the other ingredients, whisk well, pour everything into a square baking dish, introduce in the oven at 370 degrees F and bake for 20 minutes.

Cool down, slice into squares and serve.

Nutrition: calories 220, fat 2, fiber 0.5, carbs 2, protein 4

52.   Fruits Stew

Preparation time: 10 minutes

Cooking time: 10 minutes

Servings: 4

Ingredients:

1 avocado, peeled, pitted and sliced

1 cup plums, stoned and halved

2 cups water

2 teaspoons vanilla extract

1 tablespoon lemon juice

2 tablespoons stevia

Directions:

In a pan, combine the avocado with the plums, water and the other ingredients, bring to a simmer and cook over medium heat for 10 minutes.

Divide the mix into bowls and serve cold.

Nutrition: calories 178, fat 4.4, fiber 2, carbs 3, protein 5

53.   Avocado and Rhubarb Salad

Preparation time: 10 minutes

Cooking time: 0 minutes

Servings: 4

Ingredients:

1 tablespoon stevia

1 cup rhubarb, sliced and boiled

2 avocados, peeled, pitted and sliced

1 teaspoon vanilla extract

Juice of 1 lime

Directions:

In a bowl, combine the rhubarb with the avocado and the other ingredients, toss and serve.

Nutrition: calories 140, fat 2, fiber 2, carbs 4, protein 4

54.   Plums and Nuts Bowls

Preparation time: 5 minutes

Cooking time: 0 minutes

Servings: 2

Ingredients:

2 tablespoons stevia

1 cup walnuts, chopped

1 cup plums, pitted and halved

1 teaspoon vanilla extract

Directions:

In a bowl, mix the plums with the walnuts and the other ingredients, toss, divide into 2 bowls and serve cold.

Nutrition: calories 400, fat 23, fiber 4, carbs 6, protein 7

55.   Avocado and Strawberries Salad

Preparation time: 5 minutes

Cooking time: 0 minutes

Servings: 4

Ingredients:

2 avocados, pitted, peeled and cubed

1 cup strawberries, halved

Juice of 1 lime

1 teaspoon almond extract

2 tablespoons almonds, chopped

1 tablespoon stevia

Directions:

In a bowl, combine the avocados with the strawberries, and the other ingredients, toss and serve.

Nutrition: calories 150, fat 3, fiber 3, carbs 5, protein 6

56. Chocolate Watermelon Cups

Preparation time: 2 hours

Cooking time: 0 minutes

Servings: 4

Ingredients:

2 cups watermelon, peeled and cubed

1 tablespoon stevia

1 cup coconut cream

1 tablespoon cocoa powder

1 tablespoon mint, chopped

Directions:

In a blender, combine the watermelon with the stevia and the other ingredients, pulse well, divide into cups and keep in the fridge for 2 hours before serving.

Nutrition: calories 164, fat 14.6, fiber 2.1, carbs 9.9, protein 2.1

57. Vanilla Raspberries Mix

Preparation time: 10 minutes

Cooking time: 10 minutes

Servings: 4

Ingredients:

1 cup water

1 cup raspberries

3 tablespoons stevia

1 teaspoon nutmeg, ground

½ teaspoon vanilla extract

Directions:

In a pan, combine the raspberries with the water and the other ingredients, toss, cook over medium heat for 10 minutes, divide into bowls and serve.

Nutrition: calories 20, fat 0.4, fiber 2.1, carbs 4, protein 0.4

58. Ginger Cream

Preparation time: 10 minutes

Cooking time: 10 minutes

Servings: 4

Ingredients:

2 tablespoons stevia

2 cups coconut cream

1 teaspoon vanilla extract

1 tablespoon cinnamon powder

¼ tablespoon ginger, grated

Directions:

In a pan, combine the cream with the stevia and other ingredients, stir, cook over medium heat for 10 minutes, divide into bowls and serve cold.

Nutrition: calories 280, fat 28.6, fiber 2.7, carbs 7, protein 2.8

59. Chocolate Ginger Cookies

Preparation time: 10 minutes

Cooking time: 20 minutes

Servings: 6

Ingredients:

2 cups almonds, chopped

2 tablespoons flaxseed mixed with 3 tablespoons water

¼ cup avocado oil

2 tablespoons stevia

¼ cup cocoa powder

1 teaspoon baking soda

Directions:

In your food processor, combine the almonds with the flaxseed mix and the other ingredients, pulse well, scoop tablespoons out of this mix, arrange them on a lined baking sheet, flatten them a bit and cook at 360 degrees F for 20 minutes.

Serve the cookies cold.

Nutrition: calories 252, fat 41.6, fiber 6.5, carbs 11.7, protein 3

60.   Coconut Salad

Preparation time: 10 minutes

Cooking time: 0 minutes

Servings: 6

Ingredients:

2 cups coconut flesh, unsweetened and shredded

½ cup walnuts, chopped

1 cup blackberries

1 tablespoon stevia

1 tablespoon coconut oil, melted

Directions:

In a bowl, combine the coconut with the walnuts and the other ingredients, toss and serve.

Nutrition: calories 250, fat 23.8, fiber 5.8, carbs 8.9, protein 4.5

61. Mint Cookies

Preparation time: 10 minutes

Cooking time: 20 minutes

Servings: 6

Ingredients:

2 cups coconut flour

3 tablespoons flaxseed mixed with 4 tablespoons water

½ cup coconut cream

½ cup coconut oil, melted

3 tablespoons stevia

2 teaspoons mint, dried

2 teaspoons baking soda

Directions:

In a bowl, mix the coconut flour with the flaxseed, coconut cream and the other ingredients, and whisk really well.

Shape balls out of this mix, place them on a lined baking sheet, flatten them, introduce in the oven at 370 degrees F and bake for 20 minutes.

Serve the cookies cold.

Nutrition: calories 190, fat 7.32, fiber 2.2, carbs 4, protein 3

62.   Mint Avocado Bars

Preparation time: 10 minutes

Cooking time: 25 minutes

Servings: 6

Ingredients:

1 teaspoon almond extract

½ cup coconut oil, melted

2 tablespoons stevia

1 avocado, peeled, pitted and mashed

2 cups coconut flour

1 tablespoon cocoa powder

Directions:

In a bowl, combine the coconut oil with the almond extract, stevia and the other ingredients and whisk well.

Transfer this to baking pan, spread evenly, introduce in the oven and cook at 370 degrees F and bake for 25 minutes.

Cool down, cut into bars and serve.

Nutrition: calories 230, fat 12.2, fiber 4.2, carbs 15.4, protein 5.8

63.   Coconut Chocolate Cake

Preparation time: 10 minutes

Cooking time: 30 minutes

Servings: 12

Ingredients:

4 tablespoons flaxseed mixed with 5 tablespoons water

1 cup coconut flesh, unsweetened and shredded

1 teaspoon vanilla extract

2 tablespoons cocoa powder

1 teaspoon baking soda

2 cups almond flour

4 tablespoons stevia

2 tablespoons lime zest

2 cups coconut cream

Directions:

In a bowl, combine the flaxmeal with the coconut, the vanilla and the other ingredients, whisk well and transfer to a cake pan.

Cook the cake at 360 degree F for 30 minutes, cool down and serve.

Nutrition: calories 268, fat 23.9, fiber 5.1, carbs 9.4, protein 6.1

64.   Mint Chocolate Cream

Preparation time: 10 minutes

Cooking time: 0 minutes

Servings: 6

Ingredients:

1 cup coconut oil, melted

4 tablespoons cocoa powder

1 teaspoon vanilla extract

1 cup mint, chopped

2 cups coconut cream

4 tablespoons stevia

Directions:

In your food processor, combine the coconut oil with the cocoa powder, the cream and the other ingredients, pulse well, divide into bowls and serve really cold.

Nutrition: calories 514, fat 56, fiber 3.9, carbs 7.8, protein 3

65. Cranberries Cake

Preparation time: 10 minutes

Cooking time: 30 minutes

Servings: 6

Ingredients:

2 cups coconut flour

2 tablespoon coconut oil, melted

3 tablespoons stevia

1 tablespoon cocoa powder, unsweetened

2 tablespoons flaxseed mixed with 3 tablespoons water

1 cup cranberries

1 cup coconut cream

¼ teaspoon vanilla extract

½ teaspoon baking powder

Directions:

In a bowl, combine the coconut flour with the coconut oil, the stevia and the other ingredients, and whisk well.

Pour this into a cake pan lined with parchment paper, introduce in the oven and cook at 360 degrees F for 30 minutes.

Cool down, slice and serve.

Nutrition: calories 244, fat 16.7, fiber 11.8, carbs 21.3, protein 4.4

66. Sweet Zucchini Buns

Preparation time: 10 minutes

Cooking time: 30 minutes

Servings: 8

Ingredients:

1 cup almond flour

1/3 cup coconut flesh, unsweetened and shredded

1 cup zucchinis, grated

2 tablespoons stevia

1 teaspoon baking soda

½ teaspoon cinnamon powder

3 tablespoons flaxseed mixed with 4 tablespoons water

1 cup coconut cream

Directions:

In a bowl, mix the almond flour with the coconut flesh, the zucchinis and the other ingredients, stir well until you obtain a dough, shape 8 buns and arrange them on a baking sheet lined with parchment paper.

Introduce in the oven at 350 degrees and bake for 30 minutes.

Serve these sweet buns warm.

Nutrition: calories 169, fat 15.3, fiber 3.9, carbs 6.4, protein 3.2

67. Lime Custard

Preparation time: 10 minutes

Cooking time: 20 minutes

Servings: 6

Ingredients:

1 pint almond milk

4 tablespoons lime zest, grated

3 tablespoons lime juice

3 tablespoons flaxseed mixed with 4 tablespoons water

tablespoons stevia

2 teaspoons vanilla extract

Directions:

In a bowl, combine the almond milk with the lime zest, lime juice and the other ingredients, whisk well and divide into 4 ramekins.

Bake in the oven at 360 degrees F for 30 minutes.

Cool the custard down and serve.

Nutrition: calories 234, fat 21.6, fiber 4.3, carbs 9, protein 3.5

Chapter 4. Breakfast Recipes

68. Paprika Olives Spread

Preparation time: 10 minutes

Cooking time: 0 minutes

Servings: 4

Ingredients:

1 cup kalamata olives, pitted and halved

1 cup black olives, pitted and halved

1 avocado, peeled, pitted and cubed

2 scallions, chopped

2 teaspoons sweet paprika

1 tablespoon olive oil

1 tablespoon lime juice

Salt and black pepper to the taste

½ cup coconut cream

Directions:

In a blender, combine the olives with the avocado, scallions and the other ingredients, pulse well, divide into bowls and serve for breakfast.

Nutrition: calories 287, fat 27.8, fiber 6.8, carbs 12.2, protein 2.5

69.   Chives Avocado Mix

Preparation time: 5 minutes

Cooking time: 0 minutes

Servings: 4

Ingredients:

2 avocados, peeled, pitted and roughly cubed

1 tomato, cubed

1 cucumber, sliced

1 celery stalk, chopped

2 tablespoons avocado oil

1 tablespoon lime juice

Salt and black pepper to the taste

2 scallions, chopped

½ teaspoon cayenne pepper

1 tablespoon chives, chopped

Directions:

In a bowl, combine the avocados with the tomato, cucumber and the other ingredients, toss, divide between plates and serve for breakfast.

Nutrition: calories 232, fat 20.7, fiber 8, carbs 13.2, protein 2.9

70. Zucchini Pan

Preparation time: 5 minutes

Cooking time: 15 minutes

Servings: 4

Ingredients:

2 shallots, chopped

1 tablespoon olive oil

3 zucchinis, roughly cubed

2 garlic cloves, minced

2 sun-dried tomatoes, chopped

1 tablespoon capers, drained

Salt and black pepper to the taste

1 tablespoon dill, chopped

Directions:

Heat up a pan with the oil over medium heat, add the shallots, garlic and tomatoes and sauté for 5 minutes.

Add the zucchinis and the other ingredients, toss, cook over medium heat for 10 minutes more, divide between plates and serve.

Nutrition: calories 73, fat 4, fiber 2.6, carbs 9.2, protein 2.8

71. Chili Spinach and Zucchini Pan

Preparation time: 5 minutes

Cooking time: 15 minutes

Servings: 4

Ingredients:

1 pound baby spinach

1 tablespoons olive oil

2 zucchinis, sliced

1 tomato, cubed

2 shallots, chopped

1 tablespoon lime juice

2 garlic cloves, minced

2 teaspoons red chili flakes

1 teaspoon chili powder

Salt and black pepper to the taste

Directions:

Heat up a pan with the oil over medium heat, add the shallots, garlic, chili powder and chili flakes, stir and sauté for 5 minutes.

Add the spinach, zucchinis and the other ingredients, toss, cook over medium heat for 10 minutes more, divide into bowls and serve for breakfast.

Nutrition: calories 85, fat 4.3, fiber 4.1, carbs 10.6, protein 4.9

72. Basil Tomato and Cabbage Bowls

Preparation time: 5 minutes

Cooking time: 0 minutes

Servings: 4

Ingredients:

1 pound cherry tomatoes, halved

1 cup red cabbage, shredded

2 tablespoons balsamic vinegar

2 shallots, chopped

1 tablespoon avocado oil

Salt and black pepper to the taste

1 tablespoon basil, chopped

Directions:

In a bowl, combine the cabbage with the tomatoes and the other ingredients, toss and serve for breakfast.

Nutrition: calories 35, fat 0.7, fiber 2, carbs 6.6, protein 1.4

73.   Spinach and Zucchini Hash

Preparation time: 5 minutes

Cooking time: 15 minutes

Servings: 4

Ingredients:

2 zucchinis, cubed

2 cups baby spinach

A pinch of salt and black pepper

1 tablespoon olive oil

1 teaspoon chili powder

1 teaspoon rosemary, dried

½ cup coconut cream

1 tablespoon chives, chopped

Directions:

Heat up a pan with the oil over medium heat, add the zucchinis and the chili powder, stir and cook for 5 minutes.

Add the rest of the ingredients, toss, cook the mix for 10 minutes more, divide between plates and serve fro breakfast.

Nutrition: calories 121, fat 11.1, fiber 2.5, carbs 6.1, protein 2.4

74.   Tomato and Zucchini Fritters

Preparation time: 5 minutes

Cooking time: 10 minutes

Servings: 4

Ingredients:

1 pound zucchinis, grated

2 tomatoes, cubed

2 garlic cloves, minced

Salt and black pepper to the taste

1 tablespoon coconut flour

1 tablespoon flaxseed mixed with 2 tablespoons water

1 tablespoon dill, chopped

2 tablespoons olive oil

Directions:

In a bowl, mix the zucchinis with the tomatoes and the other ingredients except the oil, stir well, shape medium fritters out of this mix and flatten them

Heat up a pan with the oil over medium heat, add the fritters, cook them for 5 minutes on each side, divide between plates and serve for breakfast.

Nutrition: calories 111, fat 8.2, fiber 3.4, carbs 9, protein 2.8

75.   Peppers Casserole

Preparation time: 10 minutes

Cooking time: 25 minutes

Servings: 4

Ingredients:

1 pound mixed bell peppers, cut into strips

Salt and black pepper to the taste

4 scallions, chopped

½ teaspoon cumin, ground

½ teaspoon oregano, dried

½ teaspoon basil, dried

2 garlic cloves, minced

1 tablespoon avocado oil

2 tomatoes, cubed

1 cup cashew cheese, grated

2 tablespoons parsley, chopped

Directions:

Heat up a pan with the oil over medium heat, add the scallions and the garlic and sauté for 5 minutes.

Add the rest of the ingredients except the cheese, stir and cook for 5 minutes more.

Sprinkle the cashew cheese on top and bake everything at 380 degrees F for 15 minutes.

Divide the mix between plates and serve for breakfast.

Nutrition: calories 85, fat 3.6, fiber 3.9, carbs 11.8, protein 3.3

76. Leeks Spread

Preparation time: 5 minutes

Cooking time: 10 minutes

Servings: 4

Ingredients:

3 leeks, sliced

2 scallions, chopped

1 tablespoon avocado oil

¼ cup coconut cream

Salt and black pepper to the taste

¼ teaspoon garlic powder

½ teaspoon thyme, dried

1 tablespoon cilantro, chopped

Directions:

Heat up a pan with the oil over medium heat, add the scallions and the leeks and sauté for 5 minutes.

Add the rest of the ingredients, cook everything for 5 minutes more, blend using an immersion blender, divide into bowls and serve for breakfast.

Nutrition: calories 83, fat 4.2, fiber 2, carbs 11.3, protein 1.6

77.   Eggplant Spread

Preparation time: 10 minutes

Cooking time: 25 minutes

Servings: 4

Ingredients:

1 pound eggplants

2 tablespoons olive oil

4 spring onions, chopped

½ teaspoon chili powder

1 tablespoon lime juice

Salt and black pepper to the taste

Directions:

Arrange the eggplants in a roasting pan and bake them at 400 degrees F for 25 minutes.

Peel the eggplants, put them in a blender, add the rest of the ingredients, pulse well, divide into bowls and serve for breakfast.

Nutrition: calories 97, fat 7.3, fiber 4.6, carbs 8.9, protein 1.5

78.   Eggplant and Broccoli Casserole

Preparation time: 10 minutes

Cooking time: 35 minutes

Servings: 4

Ingredients:

1 pound eggplants, roughly cubed

1 cup broccoli florets

1 cup cashew cheese, shredded

¼ cup almond milk

2 scallions, chopped

1 tablespoon olive oil

2 tablespoons flaxseed mixed with 2 tablespoons water

1 tablespoon cilantro, chopped

Salt and black pepper to the taste

Directions:

In a roasting pan, combine the eggplants with the broccoli and the other ingredients except the cashew cheese and the almond milk and toss.

In a bowl, combine the milk with the cashew cheese, stir, pour over the eggplant mix, spread, introduce the pan in the oven and bake at 380 degrees F for 35 minutes.

Cool the casserole down, slice and serve.

Nutrition: calories 161, fat 11.4, fiber 6.6, carbs 12.8, protein 4.2

79. Creamy Avocado and Nuts Bowls

Preparation time: 5 minutes

Cooking time: 0 minutes

Servings: 4

Ingredients:

1 tablespoon walnuts, chopped

1 tablespoon pine nuts, toasted

2 avocados, peeled, pitted and roughly cubed

1 tablespoon lime juice

1 tablespoon avocado oil

Salt and black pepper to the taste

¼ cup coconut cream

Directions:

In a bowl, combine the avocados with the nuts and the other ingredients, toss, divide into smaller bowls and serve for breakfast.

Nutrition: calories 273, fat 26.3, fiber 7.5, carbs 11.1, protein 3.1

80.   Avocado and Watermelon Salad

Preparation time: 5 minutes

Cooking time: 0 minutes

Servings: 4

Ingredients:

2 cups watermelon, peeled and roughly cubed

2 avocados, peeled, pitted and roughly cubed

1 tablespoon lime juice

1 tablespoon avocado oil

¼ cup almonds, chopped

Directions:

In a bowl, combine the watermelon with the avocados and the other ingredients, toss and serve for breakfast.

Nutrition: calories 270, fat 23.1, fiber 3, carbs 16.7, protein 3.7

81. Chia and Coconut Pudding

Preparation time: 10 minutes

Cooking time: 0 minutes.

Servings: 4

Ingredients:

¼ cup walnuts, chopped

2 cups coconut milk

¼ cup coconut flakes

3 tablespoons chia seeds

1 tablespoon stevia

1 teaspoon almond extract

Directions:

In a bowl, combine the milk with the coconut flakes and the other ingredients, toss, leave aside for 10 minutes and serve for breakfast.

Nutrition: calories 414, fat 39.2, fiber 8.5, carbs 14.3, protein 7.1

82.   Tomato and Cucumber Salad

Preparation time: 5 minutes

Cooking time: 0 minutes

Servings: 4

Ingredients:

2 cups cherry tomatoes, halved

2 cucumbers, sliced

1 tablespoon lime juice

A pinch of salt and black pepper

1 tablespoon olive oil

½ cup kalamata olives, pitted and halved

1 tablespoon chives, chopped

Directions:

In a bowl, combine the tomatoes with the cucumbers and the other ingredients, toss, and serve for breakfast.

Nutrition: calories 91, fat 5.7, fiber 2.5, carbs 11, protein 2

83. Walnuts and Olives Bowls

Preparation time: 5 minutes

Cooking time: 0 minutes

Servings: 4

Ingredients:

1 cup walnuts, roughly chopped

1 cup black olives, pitted and halved

1 cup green olives, pitted and halved

1 tablespoon lime juice

1 teaspoon chili powder

1 teaspoon rosemary, dried

1 teaspoon cumin, ground

2 spring onions, chopped

1 tablespoon cilantro, chopped

A pinch of salt and black pepper

2 tablespoons avocado oil

Directions:

In a bowl, mix olives with the walnuts and the other ingredients, toss, divide into smaller bowls and serve for breakfast.

Nutrition: calories 260, fat 24, fiber 4.5, carbs 8.5, protein 8.4

84.   Kale and Broccoli Pan

Preparation time: 5 minutes

Cooking time: 12 minutes

Servings: 4

Ingredients:

1 cup broccoli florets

2 shallots, chopped

1 tablespoon olive oil

1 teaspoon sweet paprika

1 teaspoon turmeric powder

1 cup kale, torn

Salt and black pepper to the taste

¼ cup cashew cheese, grated

2 tablespoons chives, chopped

Directions:

Heat up a pan with the oil over medium heat, add the shallots and sauté for 2 minutes.

Add the broccoli, kale and the other ingredients, toss, cook for 10 minutes more, divide between plates and serve.

Nutrition: calories 63, fat 4.4, fiber 1.3, carbs 5.3, protein 1.8

85. Spinach and Berries Salad

Preparation time: 5 minutes

Cooking time: 0 minutes

Servings: 4

Ingredients:

1 cup baby spinach

1 cup blackberries

1 cup blueberries

1 tablespoon avocado oil

1 tablespoon balsamic vinegar

1 tablespoon parsley, chopped

½ cup pine nuts, chopped

Salt and black pepper to the taste

Directions:

In a salad bowl, combine the spinach with the berries and the other ingredients, toss and serve for breakfast.

Nutrition: calories 158, fat 12.4, fiber 3.8, carbs 11.5, protein 3.4

86.   Cauliflower Hash

Preparation time: 10 minutes

Cooking time: 15 minutes

Servings: 4

Ingredients:

2 cups cauliflower florets, roughly chopped

½ teaspoon basil, dried

1 teaspoon sage, dried

2 spring onions, chopped

1 tablespoon avocado oil

½ cup coconut cream

½ teaspoon sweet paprika

Salt and black pepper to the taste

1 tablespoon cilantro, chopped

Directions:

Heat up a pan with the oil over medium heat, add the onions and sauté for 5 minutes.

Add the cauliflower and the other ingredients, toss, cook everything for 10 minutes more, divide between plates and serve for breakfast.

Nutrition: calories 90, fat 7.7, fiber 2.4, carbs 5.3, protein 1.9

87. Spinach and Green Beans Casserole

Preparation time: 10 minutes

Cooking time: 40 minutes

Servings: 4

Ingredients:

1 pound green beans, trimmed and halved

4 scallions, chopped

1 tablespoon coconut oil, melted

1 cup baby spinach

2 tablespoons flaxseed mixed with 3 tablespoons water

½ cup cashew cheese, grated

Salt and black pepper to the taste

½ teaspoon thyme, chopped

Directions:

Heat up a pan with the oil over medium heat, add the scallions and sauté for 5 minutes.

Add the green beans and the other ingredients except the cheese, stir and cook for 5 minutes more.

Sprinkle the cheese on top and bake the mix at 390 degrees F for 30 minutes.

Divide the mix between plates and serve.

Nutrition: calories 273, fat 13.7, fiber 0.2, carbs 2.2, protein 1.5

88.   Spiced Zucchini and Eggplant Bowls

Preparation time: 10 minutes

Cooking time: 15 minutes

Servings: 4

Ingredients:

1 tablespoon olive oil

4 scallions, chopped

2 zucchinis, cubed

1 eggplants, cubed

1 tablespoon cilantro, chopped

1 teaspoon rosemary, dried

1 teaspoon allspice, ground

1 teaspoon nutmeg, ground

¼ cup coconut cream

Salt and black pepper to the taste

1 tablespoons chives, chopped

Directions:

Heat up a pan with the oil over medium heat, add the scallions, allspice and the nutmeg and sauté for 5 minutes.

Add the zucchini is, eggplant and the other ingredients, toss, cook over medium heat for 10 minutes, divide into bowls and serve for breakfast,

Nutrition: calories 242, fat 6.4, fiber 2, carbs 10, protein 2

Chapter 5. Lunch Recipes

89. Black Beans and Rice

Preparation time: 10 minutes

Cooking time: 30 minutes

Servings: 4

Ingredients:

3/4 cup white rice

1 medium white onion, peeled, chopped

3 1/2 cups cooked black beans

1 teaspoon minced garlic

1/4 teaspoon cayenne pepper

1 teaspoon ground cumin

1 teaspoon olive oil

1 1/2 cups vegetable broth

Directions:

Take a large pot over medium-high heat, add oil and when hot, add onion and garlic and cook for 4 minutes until saute.

Then stir in rice, cook for 2 minutes, pour in the broth, bring it to a boil, switch heat to the low level and cook for 20 minutes until tender.

Stir in remaining ingredients, cook for 2 minutes, and then serve straight away.

Nutrition:

Calories: 140 Cal

Fat: 0.9 g

Carbs: 27.1 g

Protein: 6.3 g

Fiber: 6.2 g

90. Vegetable Barley Soup

Preparation time: 5 minutes

Cooking time: 15 minutes

Servings: 8

Ingredients:

1 cup barley

14.5 ounces diced tomatoes with juice

2 large carrots, chopped

15 ounces cooked chickpeas

2 stalks celery, chopped

1 zucchini, chopped

1 medium white onion, peeled, chopped

1/2 teaspoon ground black pepper

1 teaspoon garlic powder

1 teaspoon curry powder

1 teaspoon salt

1 teaspoon paprika

1 teaspoon white sugar

1 teaspoon dried parsley

1 teaspoon Worcestershire sauce

3 bay leaves

2 quarts vegetable broth

Directions:

Place all the ingredients in a pot, stir until mixed, place it over medium-high heat and bring the mixture to a boil.

Switch heat to medium level, simmer the soup for 90 minutes until cooked, and when done, remove bay leaf from it.

Serve straight away.

Nutrition:

Calories: 188 Cal

Fat: 1.6 g

Carbs: 37 g

Protein: 7 g

Fiber: 8.4 g

91. Lentils and Rice with Fried Onions

Preparation time: 5 minutes

Cooking time: 7 minutes

Servings: 4

Ingredients:

3/4 cup long-grain white rice, cooked

1 large white onion, peeled, sliced

1 1/3 cups green lentils, cooked

½ teaspoon salt

1/4 cup vegan sour cream

¼ teaspoon ground black pepper

6 tablespoons olive oil

Directions:

Take a large skillet pan, place it over medium heat, add oil and when hot, add onions, and cook for 10 minutes until browned, set aside until required.

Take a saucepan, place it over medium heat, grease it with oil, add lentils and beans and cook for 3 minutes until warmed.

Season with salt and black pepper, cook for 2 minutes, then stir in half of the browned onions, and top with cream and remaining onions.

Serve straight away.

Nutrition:

Calories: 535 Cal

Fat: 22.1 g

Carbs: 69 g

Protein: 17.3 g

Fiber: 10.6 g

92. Asparagus Rice Pilaf

Preparation time: 10 minutes

Cooking time: 35 minutes

Servings: 4

Ingredients:

1 1/4 cups rice

1/2 pound asparagus, diced, boiled

2 ounces spaghetti, whole-grain, broken

1/4 cup minced white onion

1/2 teaspoon minced garlic

1/2 cup cashew halves

¼ teaspoon ground black pepper

½ teaspoon salt

1/4 cup vegan butter

2 1/4 cups vegetable broth

Directions:

Take a saucepan, place it over medium-low heat, add butter and when it melts, stir in spaghetti and cook for 3 minutes until golden brown.

Add onion and garlic, cook for 2 minutes until tender, then stir in rice, cook for 5 minutes, pour in the broth, season with salt and black pepper and bring it to a boil.

Switch heat to medium level, cook for 20 minutes, then add cashews and asparagus and stir until combined.

Serve straight away.

Nutrition:

Calories: 249 Cal

Fat: 10 g

Carbs: 35.1 g

Protein: 5.3 g

Fiber: 1.8 g

93.   Mexican Stuffed Peppers

Preparation time: 10 minutes

Cooking time: 40 minutes

Servings: 4

Ingredients:

2 cups cooked rice

1/2 cup chopped onion

15 ounces cooked black beans

4 large green bell peppers, destemmed, cored

1 tablespoon olive oil

1 tablespoon salt

14.5 ounce diced tomatoes

1/2 teaspoon ground cumin

1 teaspoon garlic salt

1 teaspoon red chili powder

1/2 teaspoon salt

2 cups shredded vegan Mexican cheese blend

Directions:

Boil the bell peppers in salty water for 5 minutes until softened and then set aside until required.

Heat oil over medium heat in a skillet pan, then add onion and cook for 10 minutes until softened.

Transfer the onion mixture in a bowl, add remaining ingredients, reserving ½ cup cheese blended, stir until mixed, and then fill this mixture into the boiled peppers.

Arrange the peppers in the square baking dish, sprinkle them with remaining cheese and bake for 30 minutes at 350 degrees F.

Serve straight away.

Nutrition:

Calories: 509 Cal

Fat: 22.8 g

Carbs: 55.5 g

Protein: 24 g

Fiber: 12 g

94.   Quinoa and Black Bean Chili

Preparation time: 10 minutes

Cooking time: 32 minutes

Servings: 10

Ingredients:

1 cup quinoa, cooked

38 ounces cooked black beans

1 medium white onion, peeled, chopped

1 cup of frozen corn

1 green bell pepper, deseeded, chopped

1 zucchini, chopped

1 tablespoon minced chipotle peppers in adobo sauce

1 red bell pepper, deseeded, chopped

1 jalapeno pepper, deseeded, minced

28 ounces crushed tomatoes

2 teaspoons minced garlic

1/3 teaspoon ground black pepper

¾ teaspoon salt

1 teaspoon dried oregano

1 tablespoon red chili powder

1 tablespoon ground cumin

1 tablespoon olive oil

1/4 cup chopped cilantro

Directions:

Take a large pot, place it over medium heat, add oil and when hot, add onion and cook for 5 minutes.

Then stir in garlic, cumin, and chili powder, cook for 1 minute, add remaining ingredients except for corn and quinoa, stir well and simmer for 20 minutes at medium-low heat until cooked.

Then stir in corn and quinoa, cook for 5 minutes until hot and then top with cilantro.

Serve straight away.

Nutrition:

Calories: 233 Cal

Fat: 3.5 g

Carbs: 42 g

Protein: 11.5 g

Fiber: 11.8 g

95. Mushroom Risotto

Preparation time: 10 minutes

Cooking time: 35 minutes

Servings: 4

Ingredients:

1 cup of rice

3 small white onions, peeled, chopped

1 teaspoon minced celery

1 ½ cups sliced mushrooms

½ teaspoon minced garlic

1 teaspoon minced parsley

½ teaspoon salt

¼ teaspoon ground black pepper

1 tablespoon olive oil

1 teaspoon vegan butter

¼ cup vegan cashew cream

1 cup grated vegan Parmesan cheese

1 cup of coconut milk

5 cups vegetable stock

Directions:

Take a large skillet pan, place it over medium-high heat, add oil and when hot, add onion and garlic, and cook for 5 minutes.

Transfer to a plate, add celery and parsley into the pan, stir in salt and black pepper, and cook for 3 minutes.

Then switch heat to medium-low level, stir in mushrooms, cook for 5 minutes, then pour in cream and milk, stir in rice until combined, and bring the mixture to simmer.

Pour in vegetable stock, one cup at a time until it has absorbed and, when done, stir in cheese and butter.

Serve straight away.

Nutrition:

Calories: 439 Cal

Fat: 19.5 g

Carbs: 48.7 g

Protein: 17 g

Fiber: 2 g

96.   Quinoa with Chickpeas and Tomatoes

Preparation time: 10 minutes

Cooking time: 0 minute

Servings: 6

Ingredients:

1 tomato, chopped

1 cup quinoa, cooked

½ teaspoon minced garlic

¼ teaspoon ground black pepper

½ teaspoon salt

1/2 teaspoon ground cumin

4 teaspoons olive oil

3 tablespoons lime juice

1/2 teaspoon chopped parsley

Directions:

Take a large bowl, place all the ingredients in it, except for the parsley, and stir until mixed.

Garnish with parsley and serve straight away.

Nutrition:

Calories: 185 Cal

Fat: 5.4 g

Carbs: 28.8 g

Protein: 6 g

Fiber: 4.5 g

97. Barley Bake

Preparation time: 10 minutes

Cooking time: 98 minutes

Servings: 6

Ingredients:

1 cup pearl barley

1 medium white onion, peeled, diced

2 green onions, sliced

1/2 cup sliced mushrooms

1/8 teaspoon ground black pepper

1/4 teaspoon salt

1/2 cup chopped parsley

1/2 cup pine nuts

1/4 cup vegan butter

29 ounces vegetable broth

Directions:

Place a skillet pan over medium-high heat, add butter and when it melts, stir in onion and barley, add nuts and cook for 5 minutes until light brown.

Add mushrooms, green onions and parsley, sprinkle with salt and black pepper, cook for 1 minute and then transfer the mixture into a casserole dish.

Pour in broth, stir until mixed and bake for 90 minutes until barley is tender and has absorbed all the liquid.

Serve straight away.

Nutrition:

Calories: 280 Cal

Fat: 14.2 g

Carbs: 33.2 g

Protein: 7.4 g

Fiber: 7 g

98.   Zucchini Risotto

Preparation time: 10 minutes

Cooking time: 30 minutes

Servings: 6

Ingredients:

2 cups Arborio rice

10 sun-dried tomatoes, chopped

1 medium white onion, peeled, chopped

1 tablespoon chopped basil leaves

1/2 medium zucchini, sliced

1 teaspoon dried thyme

1/3 teaspoon ground black pepper

1 tablespoon vegan butter

6 tablespoons grated vegan Parmesan cheese

7 cups vegetable broth, hot

Directions:

Take a large pot, place it over medium heat, add butter and when it melts, add onion and cook for 2 minutes.

Stir in rice, cook for another 2 minutes until toasted, and then stir in broth, 1 cup at a time until absorbed completely and creamy mixture comes together.

Then stir in remaining ingredients until combined, taste to adjust seasoning and serve.

Nutrition:

Calories: 363 Cal

Fat: 4.1 g

Carbs: 71.2 g

Protein: 9.1 g

Fiber: 3.1 g

99.   Mushroom, Lentil, and Barley Stew

Preparation time: 10 minutes

Cooking time: 6 hours

Servings: 8

Ingredients:

3/4 cup pearl barley

2 cups sliced button mushrooms

3/4 cup dry lentils

1 ounce dried shiitake mushrooms

2 teaspoons minced garlic

1/4 cup dried onion flakes

2 teaspoons ground black pepper

1 teaspoon dried basil

2 ½ teaspoons salt

2 teaspoons dried savory

3 bay leaves

2 quarts vegetable broth

Directions:

Switch on the slow cooker, place all the ingredients in it, and stir until combined.

Shut with lid and cook the stew for 6 hours at a high heat setting until cooked.

Serve straight away.

Nutrition:

Calories: 213 Cal

Fat: 1.2 g

Carbs: 44 g

Protein: 8.4 g

Fiber: 9 g

100. Tomato Barley Soup

Preparation time: 10 minutes

Cooking time: 40 minutes

Servings: 6

Ingredients:

1/4 cup barley

1 cup chopped celery

14.5 ounces peeled and diced tomatoes

1 cup chopped white onions

2 tomatoes, diced

1 cup chopped carrots

2 teaspoons minced garlic

1/8 teaspoon ground black pepper

1 teaspoon salt

2 tablespoons olive oil

2 1/2 cups water

10.75 ounces chicken broth

Directions:

Take a large saucepan, place it over medium heat, add onion, carrot, and celery, stir in garlic and cook for 10 minutes until tender.

Then add remaining ingredients, stir until combined, and bring the mixture to a boil.

Switch heat to the level, simmer the soup for 40 minutes and then serve straight away.

Nutrition:

Calories: 129 Cal

Fat: 5.5 g

Carbs: 15.3 g

Protein: 4.6 g

Fiber: 3.7 g

101. Black Beans, Corn, and Yellow Rice

Preparation time: 10 minutes

Cooking time: 25 minutes

Servings: 8

Ingredients:

8 ounces yellow rice mix

15.25 ounces cooked kernel corn

1 1/4 cups water

15 ounces cooked black beans

1 teaspoon ground cumin

2 teaspoons lime juice

2 tablespoons olive oil

Directions:

Place a saucepan over high heat, add oil, water, and rice, bring the mixture to a bowl, and then switch heat to medium-low level.

Simmer for 25 minutes until rice is tender and all the liquid has been absorbed and then transfer the rice to a large bowl.

Add remaining ingredients into the rice, stir until mixed and serve straight away.

Nutrition:

Calories: 100 Cal

Fat: 4.4 g

Carbs: 15.1 g

Protein: 2 g

Fiber: 1.4 g

102. Lemony Quinoa

Preparation time: 10 minutes

Cooking time: 0 minute

Servings: 6

Ingredients:

1 cup quinoa, cooked

1/4 of medium red onion, peeled, chopped

1 bunch of parsley, chopped

2 stalks of celery, chopped

¼ teaspoon of sea salt

1/4 teaspoon cayenne pepper

1/2 teaspoon ground cumin

1/4 cup lemon juice

1/4 cup pine nuts, toasted

Directions:

Take a large bowl, place all the ingredients in it, and stir until combined.

Serve straight away.

Nutrition:

Calories: 147 Cal

Fat: 4.8 g

Carbs: 21.4 g

Protein: 6 g

Fiber: 3 g

103. Cuban Beans and Rice

Preparation time: 10 minutes

Cooking time: 55 minutes

Servings: 6

Ingredients:

1 cup uncooked white rice

1 green bell pepper, cored, chopped

15.25 ounces cooked kidney beans

1 cup chopped white onion

4 tablespoons tomato paste

1 teaspoon minced garlic

1 teaspoon salt

1 tablespoon olive oil

2 ½ cups vegetable broth

Directions:

Take a saucepan, place it over medium heat, add oil and when hot, add onion, garlic and bell pepper and cook for 5 minutes until tender.

Then stir in salt and tomatoes, switch heat to the low level and cook for 2 minutes.

Then stir in rice and beans, pour in the broth, stir until mixed and cook for 45 minutes until rice has absorbed all the liquid.

Serve straight away.

Nutrition:

Calories: 258 Cal

Fat: 3.2 g

Carbs: 49.3 g

Protein: 7.3 g

Fiber: 5 g

104. Brown Rice, Broccoli, and Walnut

Preparation time: 5 minutes

Cooking time: 18 minutes

Servings: 4

Ingredients:

1 cup of brown rice

1 medium white onion, peeled, chopped

1 pound broccoli florets

½ cup chopped walnuts, toasted

½ teaspoon minced garlic

⅛ teaspoon ground black pepper

½ teaspoon salt

1 tablespoon vegan butter

1 cup vegetable broth

1 cup shredded vegan cheddar cheese

Directions:

Take a saucepan, place it over medium heat, add butter and when it melts, add onion and garlic and cook for 3 minutes.

Stir in rice, pour in the broth, bring the mixture to boil, then switch heat to medium-low level and simmer until rice has absorbed all the liquid.

Meanwhile, take a casserole dish, place broccoli florets in it, sprinkle with salt and black pepper, cover with a plastic wrap and microwave for 5 minutes until tender.

Place cooked rice in a dish, top with broccoli, sprinkle with nuts and cheese, and then serve.

Nutrition:

Calories: 368 Cal

Fat: 23 g

Carbs: 30.4 g

Protein: 15.1 g

Fiber: 5.7 g

105. Pecan Rice

Preparation time: 5 minutes

Cooking time: 10 minutes

Servings: 4

Ingredients:

1/4 cup chopped white onion

1/4 teaspoon ground ginger

1/2 cup chopped pecans

1/4 teaspoon salt

2 tablespoons minced parsley

1/4 teaspoon ground black pepper

1/4 teaspoon dried basil

2 tablespoons vegan margarine

1 cup brown rice, cooked

Directions:

Take a skillet pan, place it over medium heat, add margarine and when it melts, add all the ingredients except for rice and stir until mixed.

Cook for 5 minutes, then stir in rice until combined and continue cooking for 2 minutes.

Serve straight away.

Nutrition:

Calories: 280 Cal

Fat: 16.1 g

Carbs: 31 g

Protein: 4.3 g

Fiber: 3.8 g

106. Broccoli and Rice Stir Fry

Preparation time: 5 minutes

Cooking time: 10 minutes

Servings: 8

Ingredients:

16 ounces frozen broccoli florets, thawed

3 green onions, diced

½ teaspoon salt

¼ teaspoon ground black pepper

2 tablespoons soy sauce

1 tablespoon olive oil

1 ½ cups white rice, cooked

Directions:

Take a skillet pan, place it over medium heat, add broccoli, and cook for 5 minutes until tender-crisp.

Then add scallion and other ingredients, toss until well mixed and cook for 2 minutes until hot.

Serve straight away.

Nutrition:

Calories: 187 Cal

Fat: 3.4 g

Carbs: 33 g

Protein: 6.3 g

Fiber: 2.3 g

107. Lentil, Rice and Vegetable Bake

Preparation time: 10 minutes

Cooking time: 40 minutes

Servings: 6

Ingredients:

1/2 cup white rice, cooked

1 cup red lentils, cooked

1/3 cup chopped carrots

1 medium tomato, chopped

1 small onion, peeled, chopped

1/3 cup chopped zucchini

1/3 cup chopped celery

1 ½ teaspoon minced garlic

½ teaspoon ground black pepper

1 teaspoon dried basil

1 teaspoon ground cumin

1 teaspoon dried oregano

½ teaspoon salt

1 teaspoon olive oil

8 ounces tomato sauce

Directions:

Take a skillet pan, place it over medium heat, add oil and when hot, add onion and garlic, and cook for 5 minutes.

Then add remaining vegetables, season with salt, black pepper, and half of each cumin, oregano and basil and cook for 5 minutes until vegetables are tender.

Take a casserole dish, place lentils and rice in it, top with vegetables, spread with tomato sauce and sprinkle with remaining cumin, oregano, and basil, and bake for 30 minutes until bubbly.

Serve straight away.

Nutrition:

Calories: 187 Cal

Fat: 1.5 g

Carbs: 35.1 g

Protein: 9.7 g

Fiber: 8.1 g

108. Coconut Rice

Preparation time: 10 minutes

Cooking time: 25 minutes

Servings: 7

Ingredients:

2 1/2 cups white rice

1/8 teaspoon salt

40 ounces coconut milk, unsweetened

Directions:

Take a large saucepan, place it over medium heat, add all the ingredients in it and stir until mixed.

Bring the mixture to a boil, then switch heat to medium-low level and simmer rice for 25 minutes until tender and all the liquid is absorbed.

Serve straight away.

Nutrition:

Calories: 535 Cal

Fat: 33.2 g

Carbs: 57 g

Protein: 8.1 g

Fiber: 2.1 g

109. Quinoa and Chickpeas Salad

Preparation time: 10 minutes

Cooking time: 0 minute

Servings: 4

Ingredients:

3/4 cup chopped broccoli

1/2 cup quinoa, cooked

15 ounces cooked chickpeas

½ teaspoon minced garlic

1/3 teaspoon ground black pepper

2/3 teaspoon salt

1 teaspoon dried tarragon

2 teaspoons mustard

1 tablespoon lemon juice

3 tablespoons olive oil

Directions:

Take a large bowl, place all the ingredients in it, and stir until well combined. Serve straight away.

Nutrition:

Calories: 264 Cal

Fat: 12.3 g

Carbs: 32 g

Protein: 7.1 g

Fiber: 5.1 g

110. Brown Rice Pilaf

Preparation time: 5 minutes

Cooking time: 25 minutes

Servings: 4

Ingredients:

1 cup cooked chickpeas

3/4 cup brown rice, cooked

1/4 cup chopped cashews

2 cups sliced mushrooms

2 carrots, sliced

½ teaspoon minced garlic

1 1/2 cups chopped white onion

3 tablespoons vegan butter

½ teaspoon salt

¼ teaspoon ground black pepper

1/4 cup chopped parsley

Directions:

Take a large skillet pan, place it over medium heat, add butter and when it melts, add onions and cook them for 5 minutes until softened.

Then add carrots and garlic, cook for 5 minutes, add mushrooms, cook for 10 minutes until browned, add chickpeas and cook for another minute.

When done, remove the pan from heat, add nuts, parsley, salt and black pepper, toss until mixed, and garnish with parsley.

Serve straight away.

Nutrition:

Calories: 409 Cal

Fat: 17.1 g

Carbs: 54 g

Protein: 12.5 g

Fiber: 6.7 g

111. Barley and Mushrooms with Beans

Preparation time: 5 minutes

Cooking time: 15 minutes

Servings: 6

Ingredients:

1/2 cup uncooked barley

15.5 ounces white beans

1/2 cup chopped celery

3 cups sliced mushrooms

1 cup chopped white onion

1 teaspoon minced garlic

1 teaspoon olive oil

3 cups vegetable broth

Directions:

Take a saucepan, place it over medium heat, add oil and when hot, add vegetables and cook for 5 minutes until tender.

Pour in broth, stir in barley, bring the mixture to boil, and then simmer for 50 minutes until tender.

When done, add beans into the barley mixture, stir until mixed and continue cooking for 5 minutes until hot.

Serve straight away.

Nutrition:

Calories: 202 Cal

Fat: 2.1 g

Carbs: 39 g

Protein: 9.1 g

Fiber: 8.8 g

112. Vegan Curried Rice

Preparation time: 5 minutes

Cooking time: 25 minutes

Servings: 4

Ingredients:

1 cup white rice

1 tablespoon minced garlic

1 tablespoon ground curry powder

1/3 teaspoon ground black pepper

1 tablespoon red chili powder

1 tablespoon ground cumin

2 tablespoons olive oil

1 tablespoon soy sauce

1 cup vegetable broth

Directions:

Take a saucepan, place it over low heat, add oil and when hot, add garlic and cook for 3 minutes.

Then stir in all spices, cook for 1 minute until fragrant, pour in the broth, and switch heat to a high level.

Stir in soy sauce, bring the mixture to boil, add rice, stir until mixed, then switch heat to the low level and simmer for 20 minutes until rice is tender and all the liquid has absorbed.

Serve straight away.

Nutrition:

Calories: 262 Cal

Fat: 8 g

Carbs: 43 g

Protein: 5 g

Fiber: 2 g

113. Sweet Potato, Kale and Peanut Stew

Preparation time: 10 minutes

Cooking time: 45 minutes

Servings: 3

Ingredients:

1/4 cup red lentils

2 medium sweet potatoes, peeled, cubed

1 medium white onion, peeled, diced

1 cup kale, chopped

2 tomatoes, diced

1/4 cup chopped green onion

1 teaspoon minced garlic

1 inch of ginger, grated

2 tablespoons toasted peanuts

¼ teaspoon ground black pepper

1 teaspoon ground cumin

1/2 teaspoon turmeric

1/8 teaspoon cayenne pepper

1 tablespoon peanut butter

1 1/2 cups vegetable broth

2 teaspoons coconut oil

Directions:

Take a medium pot, place it medium heat, add oil and when it melts, add onions and cook for 5 minutes.

Then stir in ginger and garlic, cook for 2 minutes until fragrant, add lentils and potatoes along with all the spices, and stir until mixed.

Stir in tomatoes, pour in the broth, bring the mixture to boil, then switch heat to the low level and simmer for 30 minutes until cooked.

Then stir in peanut butter until incorporated and then puree by using an immersion blender until half-pureed.

Return stew over low heat, stir in kale, cook for 5 minutes until its leaves wilts, and then season with black pepper and salt.

Garnish the stew with peanuts and green onions and then serve.

Nutrition:

Calories: 401 Cal

Fat: 6.7 g

Carbs: 77.3 g

Protein: 10.8 g

Fiber: 16 g

114. Vegetarian Irish Stew

Preparation time: 5 minutes

Cooking time: 38 minutes

Servings: 6

Ingredients:

1 cup textured vegetable protein, chunks

½ cup split red lentils

2 medium onions, peeled, sliced

1 cup sliced parsnip

2 cups sliced mushrooms

1 cup diced celery,

1/4 cup flour

4 cups vegetable stock

1 cup rutabaga

1 bay leaf

½ cup fresh parsley

1 teaspoon sugar

¼ teaspoon ground black pepper

1/4 cup soy sauce

¼ teaspoon thyme

2 teaspoons marmite

¼ teaspoon rosemary

2/3 teaspoon salt

¼ teaspoon marjoram

Directions:

Take a large soup pot, place it over medium heat, add oil and when it gets hot, add onions and cook for 5 minutes until softened.

Then switch heat to the low level, sprinkle with flour, stir well, add remaining ingredients, stir until combined and simmer for 30 minutes until vegetables have cooked.

When done, season the stew with salt and black pepper and then serve.

Nutrition:

Calories: 117.4 Cal

Fat: 4 g

Carbs: 22.8 g

Protein: 6.5 g

Fiber: 7.3 g

115. White Bean and Cabbage Stew

Preparation time: 5 minutes

Cooking time: 8 hours

Servings: 4

Ingredients:

3 cups cooked great northern beans

1.5 pounds potatoes, peeled, cut in large dice

1 large white onion, peeled, chopped

½ head of cabbage, chopped

3 ribs celery, chopped

4 medium carrots, peeled, sliced

14.5 ounces diced tomatoes

1/3 cup pearled barley

1 teaspoon minced garlic

½ teaspoon ground black pepper

1 bay leaf

1 teaspoon dried thyme

½ teaspoon crushed rosemary

1 teaspoon salt

½ teaspoon caraway seeds

1 tablespoon chopped parsley

8 cups vegetable broth

Directions:

Switch on the slow cooker, then add all the ingredients except for salt, parsley, tomatoes, and beans and stir until mixed.

Shut the slow cooker with lid, and cook for 7 hours at low heat setting until cooked.

Then stir in remaining ingredients, stir until combined and continue cooking for 1 hour.

Serve straight away

Nutrition:

Calories: 150 Cal

Fat: 0.7 g

Carbs: 27 g

Protein: 7 g

Fiber: 9.4 g

116. Spinach and Cannellini Bean Stew

Preparation time: 10 minutes

Cooking time: 15 minutes

Servings: 6

Ingredients:

28 ounces cooked cannellini beans

24 ounces tomato passata

17 ounces spinach chopped

¼ teaspoon ground black pepper

2/3 teaspoon salt

1 ¼ teaspoon curry powder

1 cup cashew butter

¼ teaspoon cardamom

2 tablespoons olive oil

1 teaspoon salt

¼ cup cashews

2 tablespoons chopped basil

2 tablespoons chopped parsley

Directions:

Take a large saucepan, place it over medium heat, add 1 tablespoon oil and when hot, add spinach and cook for 3 minutes until fried.

Then stir in butter and tomato passata until well mixed, bring the mixture to a near boil, add beans and season with ¼ teaspoon curry powder, black pepper, and salt.

Take a small saucepan, place it over medium heat, add remaining oil, stir in cashew, stir in salt and curry powder and cook for 4 minutes until roasted, set aside until required.

Transfer cooked stew into a bowl, top with roasted cashews, basil, and parsley, and then serve.

Nutrition:

Calories: 242 Cal

Fat: 10.2 g

Carbs: 31 g

Protein: 11 g

Fiber: 8.5 g

117. Fennel and Chickpeas Provençal

Preparation time: 10 minutes

Cooking time: 50 minutes

Servings: 4

Ingredients:

15 ounces cooked chickpeas

3 fennel bulbs, sliced

1 medium onion, peeled, sliced

15 ounces diced tomatoes

10 black olives, pitted, cured

10 Kalamata olives, pitted

1 ½ teaspoon minced garlic

1 teaspoon salt

1/8 teaspoon ground black pepper

1 teaspoon Herbes de Provence

1/2 teaspoon red pepper flakes

2 tablespoons olive oil

1/2 cup water

2 tablespoons chopped parsley

Directions:

Take a saucepan, place it over medium-high heat, add oil and when hot, add onion, fennel, and garlic and cook for 20 minutes until softened.

Then add remaining ingredients except for olives and chickpeas, bring the mixture to boil, switch heat to medium-low level and simmer for 15 minutes.

Then add remaining ingredients, cook for 10 minutes until hot, garnish stew with parsley and serve.

Nutrition:

Calories: 395 Cal

Fat: 13 g

Carbs: 56 g

Protein: 16 g

Fiber: 13 g

118. Cabbage Stew

Preparation time: 10 minutes

Cooking time: 50 minutes

Servings: 6

Ingredients:

12 ounces cooked Cannellini beans

8 ounces smoked tofu, firm, sliced

1 medium cabbage, chopped

1 large white onion, peeled, julienned

2 ½ teaspoon minced garlic

1 tablespoon sweet paprika

5 tablespoons tomato paste

3 teaspoons smoked paprika

1/3 teaspoon ground black pepper

2 teaspoons dried thyme

2/3 teaspoon salt

½ tsp ground coriander

3 bay leaves

4 tablespoons olive oil

1 cup vegetable broth

Directions:

Take a large saucepan, place it over medium heat, add 3 tablespoons oil and when hot, add onion and garlic and cook for 3 minutes or until saute.

Add cabbage, pour in water, simmer for 10 minutes or until softened, then stir in all the spices and continue cooking for 30 minutes.

Add beans and tomato paste, pour in water, stir until mixed and cook for 15 minutes until thoroughly cooked.

Take a separate skillet pan, add 1 tablespoon oil and when hot, add tofu slices and cook for 5 minutes until golden brown on both sides.

Serve cooked cabbage stew with fried tofu.

Nutrition:

Calories: 182 Cal

Fat: 8.3 g

Carbs: 27 g

Protein: 5.5 g

Fiber: 9.4 g

119. Kimchi Stew

Preparation time: 10 minutes

Cooking time: 25 minutes

Servings: 4

Ingredients:

1 pound tofu, extra-firm, pressed, cut into 1-inch pieces

4 cups napa cabbage kimchi, vegan, chopped

1 small white onion, peeled, diced

2 cups sliced shiitake mushroom caps

1 ½ teaspoon minced garlic

2 tablespoons soy sauce

2 tablespoons olive oil, divided

4 cups vegetable broth

2 tablespoons chopped scallions

Directions:

Take a large pot, place it over medium heat, add 1 tablespoon oil and when hot, add tofu pieces in a single layer and cook for 10 minutes until browned on all sides.

When cooked, transfer tofu pieces to a plate, add remaining oil to the pot and when hot, add onion and cook for 5 minutes until soft.

Stir in garlic, cook for 1 minute until fragrant, stir in kimchi, continue cooking for 2 minutes, then add mushrooms and pour in broth.

Switch heat to medium-high level, bring the mixture to boil, then switch heat to medium-low level and simmer for 10 minutes until mushrooms are softened.

Stir in tofu, taste to adjust seasoning, and garnish with scallions.

Serve straight away.

Nutrition:

Calories: 153 Cal

Fat: 8.2 g

Carbs: 25 g

Protein: 8.4 g

Fiber: 2.6 g

120. African Peanut Lentil Soup

Preparation time: 10 minutes

Cooking time: 25 minutes

Servings: 3

Ingredients:

1/2 cup red lentils

1/2 medium white onion, sliced

2 medium tomatoes, chopped

1/2 cup baby spinach

1/2 cup sliced zucchini

1/2 cup sliced sweet potatoes

½ cup sliced potatoes

½ cup broccoli florets

2 teaspoons minced garlic

1 inch of ginger, grated

1 tablespoon tomato paste

1/4 teaspoon ground black pepper

1 teaspoon salt

1 ½ teaspoon ground cumin

2 teaspoons ground coriander

2 tablespoons peanuts

1 teaspoon Harissa Spice Blend

1 tablespoon sambal oelek

1/4 cup almond butter

1 teaspoon olive oil

1 teaspoon lemon juice

2 ½ cups vegetable stock

Directions:

Take a large saucepan, place it over medium heat, add oil and when hot, add onion and cook for 5 minutes until translucent.

Meanwhile, place tomatoes in a blender, add garlic, ginger and sambal oelek along with all the spices and pulse until pureed.

Pour this mixture into the onions, cook for 5 minutes, then add remaining ingredients except for spinach, peanuts and lemon juice and simmer for 15 minutes.

Taste to adjust the seasoning, stir in spinach, and cook for 5 minutes until cooked.

Ladle soup into bowls, garnish with lime juice and peanuts and serve.

Nutrition:

Calories: 411 Cal

Fat: 17 g

Carbs: 50 g

Protein: 20 g

Fiber: 18 g

121. Spicy Bean Stew

Preparation time: 5 minutes

Cooking time: 50 minutes

Servings: 4

Ingredients:

7 ounces cooked black eye beans

14 ounces chopped tomatoes

2 medium carrots, peeled, diced

7 ounces cooked kidney beans

1 leek, diced

½ a chili, chopped

1 teaspoon minced garlic

1/3 teaspoon ground black pepper

2/3 teaspoon salt

1 teaspoon red chili powder

1 lemon, juiced

3 tablespoons white wine

1 tablespoon olive oil

1 2/3 cups vegetable stock

Directions:

Take a large saucepan, place it over medium-high heat, add oil and when hot, add leeks and cook for 8 minutes or until softened.

Then add carrots, continue cooking for 4 minutes, stir in chili and garlic, pour in the wine, and continue cooking for 2 minutes.

Add tomatoes, stir in lemon juice, pour in the stock and bring the mixture to boil.

Switch heat to medium level, simmer for 35 minutes until stew has thickened, then add both beans along with remaining ingredients and cook for 5 minutes until hot.

Serve straight away.

Nutrition:

Calories: 114 Cal

Fat: 1.6 g

Carbs: 19 g

Protein: 6 g

Fiber: 8.4 g

122. Eggplant, Onion and Tomato Stew

Preparation time: 5 minutes

Cooking time: 5 minutes

Servings: 4

Ingredients:

3 1/2 cups cubed eggplant

1 cup diced white onion

2 cups diced tomatoes

1 teaspoon ground cumin

1/8 teaspoon ground cayenne pepper

1 teaspoon salt

1 cup tomato sauce

1/2 cup water

Directions:

Switch on the instant pot, place all the ingredients in it, stir until mixed, and seal the pot.

Press the 'manual' button and cook for 5 minutes at high-pressure setting until cooked.

When done, do quick pressure release, open the instant pot, and stir the stew.

Serve straight away.

Nutrition:

Calories: 88 Cal

Fat: 1 g

Carbs: 21 g

Protein: 3 g

Fiber: 6 g

123. White Bean Stew

Preparation time: 5 minutes

Cooking time: 10 hours and 10 minutes

Servings: 10

Ingredients:

2 cups chopped spinach

28 ounces diced tomatoes

2 pounds white beans, dried

2 cups chopped chard

2 large carrots, peeled, diced

2 cups chopped kale

3 large celery stalks, diced

1 medium white onion, peeled, diced

1 ½ teaspoon minced garlic

2 tablespoons salt

1 teaspoon dried rosemary

½ teaspoon Ground black pepper, to taste

1 teaspoon dried thyme

1 teaspoon dried oregano

1 bay leaf

10 cups water

Directions:

Switch on the slow cooker, add all the ingredients in it, except for kale, chard, and spinach and stir until combined.

Shut the cooker with lid and cook for 10 hours at a low heat setting until thoroughly cooked.

When done, stir in kale, chard, and spinach, and cook for 10 minutes until leaves wilt.

Serve straight away.

Nutrition:

Calories: 109 Cal

Fat: 2.4 g

Carbs: 17.8 g

Protein: 5.3 g

Fiber: 6 g

124. Brussel Sprouts Stew

Preparation time: 10 minutes

Cooking time: 55 minutes

Servings: 4

Ingredients:

35 ounces Brussels sprouts

5 medium potato, peeled, chopped

1 medium onion, peeled, chopped

2 carrot, peeled, cubed

2 teaspoon smoked paprika

1/8 teaspoon ground black pepper

1/8 teaspoon salt

3 tablespoons caraway seeds

1/2 teaspoon red chili powder

1 tablespoon nutmeg

1 tablespoon olive oil

4 ½ cups hot vegetable stock

Directions:

Take a large pot, place it over medium-high heat, add oil and when hot, add onion and cook for 1 minute.

Then add carrot and potato, cook for 2 minutes, then add Brussel sprouts and cook for 5 minutes.

Stir in all the spices, pour in vegetable stock, bring the mixture to boil, switch heat to medium-low and simmer for 45 minutes until cooked and stew reach to desired thickness.

Serve straight away.

Nutrition:

Calories: 156 Cal

Fat: 3 g

Carbs: 22 g

Protein: 12 g

Fiber: 5.1100 g

125. Vegetarian Gumbo

Preparation time: 10 minutes

Cooking time: 45 minutes

Servings: 4

Ingredients:

1 1/2 cups diced zucchini

16-ounces cooked red beans

4 cups sliced okra

1 1/2 cups diced green pepper

1 1/2 cups chopped white onion

1 1/2 cups diced red bell pepper

8 cremini mushrooms, quartered

1 cup sliced celery

3 teaspoons minced garlic

1 medium tomato, chopped

1 teaspoon red pepper flakes

1 teaspoon dried thyme

3 tablespoons all-purpose flour

1 tablespoon smoked paprika

1 teaspoon dried oregano

1/4 teaspoon nutmeg

1 teaspoon soy sauce

1 1/2 teaspoons liquid smoke

2 tablespoons mustard

1 tablespoon apple cider vinegar

1 tablespoon Worcestershire sauce, vegetarian

1/2 teaspoon hot sauce

3 tablespoons olive oil

4 cups vegetable stock

1/2 cups sliced green onion

4 cups cooked jasmine rice

Directions:

Take a Dutch oven, place it over medium heat, add oil and flour and cook for 5 minutes until fragrant.

Switch heat to the medium low level, and continue cooking for 20 minutes until roux becomes dark brown, whisking constantly.

Meanwhile, place the tomato in a food processor, add garlic and onion along with remaining ingredients, except for stock, zucchini, celery, mushroom, green and red bell pepper, and pulse for 2 minutes until smooth.

Pour the mixture into the pan, return pan over medium-high heat, stir until mixed, and cook for 5 minutes until all the liquid has evaporated.

Stir in stock, bring it to simmer, then add remaining vegetables and simmer for 20 minutes until tender.

Garnish gumbo with green onions and serve with rice.

Nutrition:

Calories: 160 Cal

Fat: 7.3 g

Carbs: 20 g

Protein: 7 g

Fiber: 5.7 g

126. Black Bean and Quinoa Stew

Preparation time: 10 minutes

Cooking time: 6 hours

Servings: 6

Ingredients:

1 pound black beans, dried, soaked overnight

3/4 cup quinoa, uncooked

1 medium red bell pepper, cored, chopped

1 medium red onion, peeled, diced

1 medium green bell pepper, cored, chopped

28-ounce diced tomatoes

2 dried chipotle peppers

1 ½ teaspoon minced garlic

2/3 teaspoon sea salt

2 teaspoons red chili powder

1/3 teaspoon ground black pepper

1 teaspoon coriander powder

1 dried cinnamon stick

1/4 cup cilantro

7 cups of water

Directions:

Switch on the slow cooker, add all the ingredients in it, except for salt, and stir until mixed.

Shut the cooker with lid and cook for 6 hours at a high heat setting until cooked.

When done, stir salt into the stew until mixed, remove cinnamon sticks and serve.

Nutrition:

Calories: 308 Cal

Fat: 2 g

Carbs: 70 g

Protein: 23 g

Fiber: 32 g

127. Root Vegetable Stew

Preparation time: 10 minutes

Cooking time: 8 hours and 10 minutes

Servings: 6

Ingredients:

2 cups chopped kale

1 large white onion, peeled, chopped

1 pound parsnips, peeled, chopped

1 pound potatoes, peeled, chopped

2 celery ribs, chopped

1 pound butternut squash, peeled, deseeded, chopped

1 pound carrots, peeled, chopped

3 teaspoons minced garlic

1 pound sweet potatoes, peeled, chopped

1 bay leaf

1 teaspoon ground black pepper

1/2 teaspoon sea salt

1 tablespoon chopped sage

3 cups vegetable broth

Directions:

Switch on the slow cooker, add all the ingredients in it, except for the kale, and stir until mixed.

Shut the cooker with lid and cook for 8 hours at a low heat setting until cooked.

When done, add kale into the stew, stir until mixed, and cook for 10 minutes until leaves have wilted.

Serve straight away.

Nutrition:

Calories: 120 Cal

Fat: 1 g

Carbs: 28 g

Protein: 4 g

Fiber: 6 g

128. Portobello Mushroom Stew

Preparation time: 10 minutes

Cooking time: 8 hours

Servings: 4

Ingredients:

8 cups vegetable broth

1 cup dried wild mushrooms

1 cup dried chickpeas

3 cups chopped potato

2 cups chopped carrots

1 cup corn kernels

2 cups diced white onions

1 tablespoon minced parsley

3 cups chopped zucchini

1 tablespoon minced rosemary

1 1/2 teaspoon ground black pepper

1 teaspoon dried sage

2/3 teaspoon salt

1 teaspoon dried oregano

3 tablespoons soy sauce

1 1/2 teaspoons liquid smoke

8 ounces tomato paste

Directions:

Switch on the slow cooker, add all the ingredients in it, and stir until mixed.

Shut the cooker with lid and cook for 10 hours at a high heat setting until cooked.

Serve straight away.

Nutrition:

Calories: 447 Cal

Fat: 36 g

Carbs: 24 g

Protein: 11 g

Fiber: 2 g

Chapter 6. Dinner Recipes

129. Tofu Fajita Bowl

Preparation Time: 5minutes

Cooking Time: 10minutes

Servings: 4

Ingredients:

2 tbsp olive oil

1½ lb tofu, cut into strips

Salt and ground black pepper to taste

2 tbsp Tex-Mex seasoning

1 small iceberg lettuce, chopped

2 large tomatoes, deseeded and chopped

2 avocados, halved, pitted, and chopped

1 green bell pepper, deseeded and thinly sliced

1 yellow onion, thinly sliced

4 tbsp fresh cilantro leaves

½ cup shredded dairy- free parmesan cheese blend

1 cup plain unsweetened yogurt

Directions:

Heat the olive oil in a medium skillet over medium heat, season the tofu with salt, black pepper, and Tex-Mex seasoning. Fry in the oil on both sides until golden and cooked, 5 to 10 minutes. Transfer to a plate.

Divide the lettuce into 4 serving bowls, share the tofu on top, and add the tomatoes, avocados, bell pepper, onion, cilantro, and cheese.

Top with dollops of plain yogurt and serve immediately with low carb tortillas.

Nutrition:

Calories:263, Total Fat:26.4g, Saturated Fat:8.8g, Total Carbs:4g, Dietary Fiber:1g, Sugar:3g, Protein:4g, Sodium:826mg

130. Indian Style Tempeh Bake

Preparation Time: 10minutes

Cooking Time: 26minutes

Servings: 4

Ingredients:

3 tbsp unsalted butter

6 tempeh, cut into 1-inch cubes

Salt and ground black pepper to taste

2 ½ tbsp garam masala

1 cup baby spinach, tightly pressed

1¼ cups coconut cream

1 tbsp fresh cilantro, finely chopped

Directions:

Preheat the oven to 350 F and grease a baking dish with cooking spray. Set aside.

Heat the ghee in a medium skillet over medium heat, season the tempeh with salt and black pepper, and cook in the oil on both sides until golden on the outside, 6 minutes.

Mix in half of the garam masala and transfer the tempeh (with juicesinto the baking dish.

Add the spinach, and spread the coconut cream on top. Bake in the oven for 20 minutes or until the cream is bubbly.

Remove the dish, garnish with cilantro, and serve with cauliflower couscous.

Nutrition:

Calories:598, Total Fat:56g, Saturated Fat:18.8g, Total Carbs12:g, Dietary Fiber:3g, Sugar:5g, Protein:15g, Sodium:762mg

131. Tofu- Seitan Casserole

Preparation Time: 10minutes

Cooking Time: 20minutes

Servings: 4

Ingredients:

1 tofu, shredded

7 oz seitan, chopped

8 oz dairy- free cream cheese (vegan

1 tbsp Dijon mustard

1 tbsp plain vinegar

10 oz shredded cheddar cheese

Salt and ground black pepper to taste

Directions:

Preheat the oven to 350 F and grease a baking dish with cooking spray. Set aside.

Spread the tofu and seitan in the bottom of the dish.

In a small bowl, mix the cashew cream, Dijon mustard, vinegar, and two-thirds of the cheddar cheese. Spread the mixture on top of the tofu and seitan, season with salt and black pepper, and cover with the remaining cheese.

Bake in the oven for 15 to 20 minutes or until the cheese melts and is golden brown.

Remove the dish and serve with steamed collards.

Nutrition:

Calories475:, Total Fat:41.2g, Saturated Fat:12.3g, Total Carbs:6g, Dietary Fiber:3g, Sugar:2g, Protein:24g, Sodium:755mg

132. Ginger Lime Tempeh

Preparation Time: 10 minutes

Cooking Time: 40 minutes

Servings: 4

Ingredients:

5 kaffir lime leaves

1 tbsp cumin powder

1 tbsp ginger powder

1 cup plain unsweetened yogurt

2 lb tempeh

Salt and ground black pepper to taste

1 tbsp olive oil

2 limes, juiced

Directions:

In a large bowl, combine the kaffir lime leaves, cumin, ginger, and plain yogurt. Add the tempeh, season with salt, and black pepper, and mix to coat well. Cover the bowl with a plastic wrap and marinate in the refrigerator for 2 to 3 hours.

Preheat the oven to 350 F and grease a baking sheet with cooking spray.

Take out the tempeh and arrange on the baking sheet. Drizzle with olive oil, lime juice, cover with aluminum foil, and slow-cook in the oven for 1 to 1 ½ hours or until the tempeh cooks within.

Remove the aluminum foil, turn the broiler side of the oven on, and brown the top of the tempeh for 5 to 10 minutes.

Take out the tempeh and serve warm with red cabbage slaw.

Nutrition:

Calories:285, Total Fat:25.6g, Saturated Fat:13.6g, Total Carbs:7g, Dietary Fiber:2g, Sugar:2g, Protein:11g, Sodium:772mg

133. Tofu Mozzarella

Preparation Time: 10minutes

Cooking Time: 35minutes

Servings: 4

Ingredients:

1½ lb tofu, halved lengthwise

Salt and ground black pepper to taste

2 eggs

2 tbsp Italian seasoning

1 pinch red chili flakes

½ cup sliced Pecorino Romano cheese

¼ cup fresh parsley, chopped

4 tbsp butter

2 garlic cloves, minced

2 cups crushed tomatoes

1 tbsp dried basil

Salt and ground black pepper to taste

½ lb sliced mozzarella cheese

Directions:

Preheat the oven to 400 F and grease a baking dish with cooking spray. Set aside.

Season the tofu with salt and black pepper; set aside.

In a medium bowl, whisk the eggs with the Italian seasoning, and red chili flakes. In a plate, combine the Pecorino Romano cheese with parsley.

Melt the butter in a medium skillet over medium heat.

Quickly dip the tofu in the egg mixture and then dredge generously in the cheese mixture. Place in the butter and fry on both sides until the cheese melts and is golden brown, 8 to 10 minutes. Place on a plate and set aside.

Sauté the garlic in the same pan and mix in the tomatoes. Top with the basil, salt, and black pepper, and cook for 5 to 10 minutes. Pour the sauce into the baking dish.

Lay the tofu pieces in the sauce and top with the mozzarella cheese. Bake in the oven for 10 to 15 minutes or until the cheese melts completely.

Remove the dish and serve with leafy green salad.

Nutrition:

Calories:140, Total Fat:13.2g, Saturated Fat:7.1g, Total Carbs:2g, Dietary Fiber:0g, Sugar:0g, Protein:3g, Sodium:78mg1

134. Seitan Meatza with Kale

Preparation Time: 10minutes

Cooking Time: 22minutes

Servings: 4

Ingredients:

1 lb ground seitan

Salt and black pepper to taste

2 cups powdered Parmesan cheese

¼ tsp onion powder

¼ tsp garlic powder

½ cup unsweetened tomato sauce

1 tsp white vinegar

½ tsp liquid smoke

¼ cup baby kale, chopped roughly

1 cup mozzarella cheese

Directions:

Preheat the oven to 400 F and line a medium pizza pan with parchment paper and grease with cooking spray. Set aside.

In a medium bowl, combine the seitan, salt, black pepper, and parmesan cheese. Spread the mixture on the pizza pan to fit the shape of the pan. Bake in the oven for 15 minutes or until the meat cooks.

Meanwhile in a medium bowl, mix the onion powder, garlic powder, tomato sauce, vinegar, and liquid smoke. Remove the meat crust from the oven and spread the tomato mixture on top. Add the kale and sprinkle with the mozzarella cheese.

Bake in the oven for 7 minutes or until the cheese melts.

Take out from the oven, slice, and serve warm.

Nutrition:

Calories:601, Total Fat:51.8g, Saturated Fat:16.4g, Total Carbs:18g, Dietary Fiber:5g, Sugar:3g, Protein:23g, Sodium:398mg

135. Taco Tempeh Casserole

Preparation Time: 10minutes

Cooking Time: 20minutes

Servings: 4

Ingredients:

1 Tempeh, shredded

1/3 cup vegan mayonnaise

8 oz dairy- free cream cheese (vegan

1 yellow onion, sliced

1 yellow bell pepper, deseeded and chopped

2 tbsp taco seasoning

½ cup shredded cheddar cheese

Salt and ground black pepper to taste

Directions:

Preheat the oven to 400 F and grease a baking dish with cooking spray.

Into the dish, put the tempeh, mayonnaise, cashew cream, onion, bell pepper, taco seasoning, and two-thirds of the cheese, salt, and black pepper. Mix the Ingredients and top with the remaining cheese.

Bake in the oven for 15 to 20 minutes or until the cheese melts and is golden brown.

Remove the dish, plate, and serve with lettuce leaves.

Nutrition:

Calories:132, Total Fat:11.5g, Saturated Fat4:4.3g, Total Carbs:7g, Dietary Fiber:4g, Sugar:2g, Protein:1g, Sodium:10mg

136. Broccoli Tempeh Alfredo

Preparation Time: 10minutes

Cooking Timee: 15minutes

Servings: 4

Ingredients:

6 slices tempeh, chopped

2 tbsp butter

4 tofu, cut into 1-inch cubes

Salt and ground black pepper to taste

4 garlic cloves, minced

1 cup baby kale, chopped

1 ½ cups full- fat heavy cream

1 medium head broccoli, cut into florets

¼ cup shredded parmesan cheese

Directions:

Put the tempeh in a medium skillet over medium heat and fry until crispy and brown, 5 minutes. Spoon onto a plate and set aside.

Melt the butter in the same skillet, season the tofu with salt and black pepper, and cook on both sides until goldern- brown. Spoon onto the tempeh's plate and set aside.

Add the garlic to the skillet, sauté for 1 minute.

Mix in the full- fat heavy cream, tofu, and tempeh, and kale, allow simmering for 5 minutes or until the sauce thickens.

Meanwhile, pour the broccoli into a large safe-microwave bowl, sprinkle with some water, season with salt, and black pepper, and microwave for 2 minutes or until the broccoli softens.

Spoon the broccoli into the sauce, top with the parmesan cheese, stir and cook until the cheese melts. Turn the heat off.

Spoon the mixture into a serving platter and serve warm.

Nutrition:

Calories:193, Total Fat:20.1g, Saturated Fat:12.5g, Total Carbs:3g, Dietary Fiber:0g, Sugar:2g, Protein:1g, Sodium:100mg

137. Avocado Seitan

Preparation Time: 10 minutes

Cooking Time: 2 hours 15 minutes

Servings: 4

Ingredients:

1 white onion, finely chopped

¼ cup vegetable stock

3 tbsp coconut oil

3 tbsp tamari sauce

3 tbsp chili pepper

1 tbsp red wine vinegar

Salt and ground black pepper to taste

2 lb Seitan

1 large avocado, halved and pitted

½ lemon, juiced

Directions:

In a large pot, combine the onion, vegetable stock, coconut oil, tamari sauce, chili pepper, red wine vinegar, salt, black pepper. Add the seitan, close the lid, and cook over low heat for 2 hours.

Scoop the avocado pulp into a bowl, add the lemon juice, and using a fork, mash the avocado into a puree. Set aside.

When ready, turn the heat off and mix in the avocado. Adjust the taste with salt and black pepper.

Spoon onto a serving platter and serve warm.

Nutrition:

Calories:412, Total Fat:43g, Saturated Fat:37g, Total Carbs:9g, Dietary Fiber:3g, Sugar:0g, Protein:5g, Sodium:12mg

138. Seitan Mushroom Burgers

Preparation Time: 15 minutes

Cooking Time: 13 minutes

Servings: 4

Ingredients:

1 ½ lb ground seitan

Salt and ground black pepper to taste

1 tbsp unsweetened tomato sauce

6 large Portobello caps, destemmed

1 tbsp olive oil

6 slices cheddar cheese

For topping:

4 lettuce leaves

4 large tomato slices

¼ cup mayonnaise

Directions:

In a medium bowl, combine the seitan, salt, black pepper, and tomato sauce. Using your hands, mold the mixture into 4 patties, and set aside.

Rinse the mushrooms under running water and pat dry.

Heat the olive oil in a medium skillet; place in the Portobello caps and cook until softened, 3 to 4 minutes. Transfer to a serving plate and set aside.

Put the seitan patties in the skillet and fry on both sides until brown and compacted, 8 minutes. Place the vegan cheddar slices on the food, allow melting for 1 minute and lift each patty onto each mushroom cap.

Divide the lettuce on top, then the tomato slices, and add some mayonnaise.

Serve immediately.

Nutrition:

Calories:304, Total Fat:29g, Saturated Fat:23.5g, Total Carbs:8g, Dietary Fiber:3g, Sugar:1g, Protein:8g, Sodium:8mg

139. Taco Tempeh Stuffed Peppers

Preparation Time: 15 minutes

Cooking Time: 41 minutes

Servings: 6

Ingredients:

6 yellow bell peppers, halved and deseeded

1 ½ tbsp olive oil

Salt and ground black pepper to taste

3 tbsp butter

3 garlic cloves, minced

½ white onion, chopped

2 lbs. ground tempeh

3 tsp taco seasoning

1 cup riced broccoli

¼ cup grated cheddar cheese

Plain unsweetened yogurt for serving

Directions:

Preheat the oven to 400 F and grease a baking dish with cooking spray. Set aside.

Drizzle the bell peppers with the olive oil and season with some salt. Set aside.

Melt the butter in a large skillet and sauté the garlic and onion for 3 minutes. Stir in the tempeh, taco seasoning, salt, and black pepper. Cook until the meat is no longer pink, 8 minutes.

Mix in the broccoli until adequately incorporated. Turn the heat off.

Spoon the mixture into the peppers, top with the cheddar cheese, and place the peppers in the baking dish. Bake in the oven until the cheese melts and is bubbly, 30 minutes.

Remove the dish from the oven and plate the peppers. Top with the palin yogurt and serve warm.

Nutrition:

Calories:251, Total Fat:22.5g, Saturated Fat:3.8g, Total Carbs:13g, Dietary Fiber:9g, Sugar:2g, Protein:3g, Sodium:23mg

140. Tangy Tofu Meatloaf

Preparation Time: 10 minutes

Cooking Time: 40 minutes

Servings: 6

Ingredients:

2 ½ lb ground tofu

Salt and ground black pepper to taste

3 tbsp flaxseed meal

2 large eggs

2 tbsp olive oil

1 lemon,1 tbsp juiced

¼ cup freshly chopped parsley

¼ cup freshly chopped oregano

4 garlic cloves, minced

Lemon slices to garnish

Directions:

Preheat the oven to 400 F and grease a loaf pan with cooking spray. Set aside.

In a large bowl, combine the tofu, salt, black pepper, and flaxseed meal. Set aside.

In a small bowl, whisk the eggs with the olive oil, lemon juice, parsley, oregano, and garlic. Pour the mixture onto the mix and combine well.

Spoon the tofu mixture into the loaf pan and press to fit into the pan. Bake in the middle rack of the oven for 30 to 40 minutes.

Remove the pan, tilt to drain the meat's liquid, and allow cooling for 5 minutes.

Slice, garnish with some lemon slices and serve with braised green beans.

Nutrition:

Calories:238, Total Fat:26.3g, Saturated Fat:14.9g, Total Carbs:1g, Dietary Fiber:0g, Sugar:0g, Protein:1g, Sodium:183mg

141. Vegan Bacon Wrapped Tofu with Buttered Spinach

Preparation Time: 5 minutes

Cooking Time: 20 minutes

Servings: 4

Ingredients:

For the bacon wrapped tofu:

4 tofu

8 slices vegan bacon

Salt and black pepper to taste

2 tbsp olive oil

For the buttered spinach:

2 tbsp butter

1 lb spinach

4 garlic cloves

Salt and ground black pepper to taste

Directions:

For the bacon wrapped tofu:

Preheat the oven to 450 F.

Wrap each tofu with two vegan bacon slices, season with salt and black pepper, and place on the baking sheet. Drizzle with the olive oil and bake in the oven for 15 minutes or until the vegan bacon browns and the tofu cooks within.

For the buttered spinach:

Meanwhile, melt the butter in a large skillet, add and sauté the spinach and garlic until the leaves wilt, 5 minutes. Season with salt and black pepper.

Remove the tofu from the oven and serve with the buttered spinach.

Nutrition:

Calories:260, Total Fat:24.7g, Saturated Fat:14.3g, Total Carbs:4g, Dietary Fiber:0g, Sugar:2g, Protein:6g, Sodium:215mg

142. Seitan Zoodle Bowl

Preparation Time: 15 minutes

Cooking Time: 13 minutes

Servings: 4

Ingredients:

5 garlic cloves, minced, divided

¼ tsp pureed onion

Salt and ground black pepper to taste

2 ½ lb Seitan, cut into strips

2 tbsp avocado oil

3 large eggs, lightly beaten

¼ cup vegetable broth

2 tbsp coconut aminos

1 tbsp white vinegar

½ cup freshly chopped scallions

1 tsp red chili flakes

4 medium zucchinis, spiralized

½ cup toasted pine nuts, for topping

Directions:

In a medium bowl, combine the half of the pureed garlic, onion, salt, and black pepper. Add the seitan and mix well.

Heat the avocado oil in a large, deep skillet over medium heat and add the seitan. Cook for 8 minutes. Transfer to a plate.

Pour the eggs into the pan and scramble for 1 minute. Spoon the eggs to the side of the seitan and set aside.

Reduce the heat to low and in a medium bowl, mix the vegetable broth, coconut aminos, vinegar, scallions, remaining garlic, and red chili flakes. Mix well and simmer for 3 minutes.

Stir in the seitan, zucchini, and eggs. Cook for 1 minute and turn the heat off. Adjust the taste with salt and black pepper.

Spoon the zucchini food into serving plates, top with the pine nuts and serve warm.

Nutrition:

Calories:687, Total Fat:54.5g, Saturated Fat:27.4g, Total Carbs:9g, Dietary Fiber:2g, Sugar:4g, Protein:38g, Sodium:883mg

143. Tofu Parsnip Bake

Preparation Time: 5 minutes

Cooking Time: 44 minutes

Servings: 4

Ingredients:

6 vegan bacon slices, chopped

2 tbsp butter

½ lb parsnips, peeled and diced

2 tbsp olive oil

1 lb ground tofu

Salt and ground black pepper to taste

2 tbsp butter

1 cup full- fat heavy cream

2 oz dairy- free cream cheese (vegan), softened

1 ¼ cups grated cheddar cheese

¼ cup chopped scallions

Directions:

Preheat the oven to 300 F and lightly grease a baking dish with cooking spray. Set aside.

Put the vegan bacon in a medium pot and fry on both sides until brown and crispy, 7 minutes. Spoon onto a plate and set aside.

Melt the butter in a large skillet and sauté the parsnips until softened and lightly browned. Transfer to the baking sheet and set aside.

Heat the olive oil in the same pan and cook the tofu (seasoned with salt and black pepper). Spoon onto a plate and set aside too.

Add the butter, full- fat heavy cream, cashew cream, two-thirds of the cheddar cheese, salt, and black pepper to the pot. Melt the Ingredients over medium heat with frequent stirring, 7 minutes.

Spread the parsnips in the baking dish, top with the tofu, pour the full- fat heavy cream mixture over, and scatter the top with the vegan bacon and scallions.

Sprinkle the remaining cheese on top, and bake in the oven until the cheese melts and is golden, 30 minutes.

Remove the dish, spoon the food into serving plates, and serve immediately.

Nutrition:

Calories:534, Total Fat:56g, Saturated Fat:34.6g, Total Carbs:4g, Dietary Fiber:1g, Sugar:1g, Protein:7g, Sodium:430mg

144. Squash Tempeh Lasagna

Preparation Time: 15 minutes

Cooking Time: 40 minutes

Servings: 4

Ingredients:

2 tbsp butter

1 ½ lb ground tempeh

Salt and ground black pepper to taste

1 tsp garlic powder

1 tsp onion powder

2 tbsp coconut flour

1 ½ cup grated mozzarella cheese

1/3 cup parmesan cheese

2 cups crumbled cottage cheese

1 large egg, beaten into a bowl

2 cups unsweetened marinara sauce

1 tbsp dried Italian mixed herbs

¼ tsp red chili flakes

4 large yellow squash, sliced

¼ cup fresh basil leaves

Directions:

Preheat the oven to 375 F and grease a baking dish with cooking spray. Set aside.

Melt the butter in a large skillet over medium heat and cook the tempeh until brown, 10 minutes. Set aside to cool.

In a medium bowl, mix the garlic powder, onion powder, coconut flour, salt, black pepper, mozzarella cheese, half of the parmesan cheese, cottage cheese, and egg. Set aside.

In another bowl, combine the marinara sauce, mixed herbs, and red chili flakes. Set aside.

Make a single layer of the squash slices in the baking dish; spread a quarter of the egg mixture on top, a layer of the tempeh, then a quarter of the marinara sauce. Repeat the layering process in the same ingredient proportions and sprinkle the top with the remaining parmesan cheese.

Bake in the oven until golden brown on top, 30 minutes.

Remove the dish from the oven, allow cooling for 5 minutes, garnish with the basil leaves, slice and serve.

Nutrition:

Calories:194, Total Fat:17.4g, Saturated Fat:2.1g, Total Carbs:7g, Dietary Fiber:3g, Sugar:2g, Protein:7g, Sodium:72mg

145. Bok Choy Tofu Skillet

Preparation Time: 10 minutes

Cooking Time: 18 minutes

Servings: 4

Ingredients:

2 lb tofu, cut into 1-inch cubes

Salt and ground black pepper to taste

4 vegan bacon slices, chopped

1 tbsp coconut oil

1 orange bell pepper, deseeded, cut into chunks

2 cups baby bok choy

2 tbsp freshly chopped oregano

2 garlic cloves, pressed

Directions:

Season the tofu with salt and black pepper, and set aside.

Heat a large skillet over medium heat and fry the vegan bacon until brown and crispy. Transfer to a plate.

Melt the coconut oil in the skillet and cook the tofu until golden- brown and cooked through, 10 minutes. Remove onto the vegan bacon plate and set aside.

Add the bell pepper and bok choy to the skillet and sauté until softened, 5 minutes. Stir in the vegan bacon, tofu, oregano, and garlic. Season with salt and black pepper and cook for 3 minutes or until the flavors incorporate. Turn the heat off.

Plate the dish and serve with cauliflower rice.

Nutrition:

Calories:273, Total Fat:18.7g, Saturated Fat:7.9g, Total Carbs:15g, Dietary Fiber:4g, Sugar:8g, Protein:15g, Sodium:341mg

146. Quorn Sausage Frittata

Preparation Time: 10 minutes

Cooking Time: 33 minutes

Servings: 4

Ingredients:

12 whole eggs

1 cup plain unsweetened yogurt

Salt and ground black pepper to taste

1 tbsp butter

1 celery stalk, chopped

12 oz quorn sausages

¼ cup shredded cheddar cheese

Directions:

Preheat the oven to 350 F.

In a medium bowl, whisk the eggs, plain yogurt, salt, and black pepper.

Melt the butter in a large (safe ovenskillet over medium heat. Sauté the celery until soft, 5 minutes. Transfer the celery into a plate and set aside.

Add the quorn sausages to the skillet and cook until brown with frequent stirring to break the lumps that form, 8 minutes.

Flatten the quorn sausage in the bottom of the skillet using the spoon, scatter the celery on top, pour the egg mixture all over, and sprinkle with the cheddar cheese.

Put the skillet in the oven and bake until the eggs set and cheese melts, 20 minutes.

Remove the skillet, slice the frittata, and serve warm with kale salad.

Nutrition:

Calories:293, Total Fat:27.9g, Saturated Fat:2.9g, Total Carbs:11g, Dietary Fiber:4g, Sugar:2g, Protein:5g, Sodium:20mg

147. Jamaican Jerk Tempeh

Preparation Time: 15 minutes

Cooking Time: 45 minutes

Servings: 4

Ingredients:

½ cup plain unsweetened yogurt

2 tbsp melted butter

2 tbsp Jamaican jerk seasoning

Salt and black pepper to taste

2 lb tempeh

3 tbsp tofu

¼ cup almond meal

Directions:

Preheat the oven to 350 F and grease a baking sheet with cooking spray.

In a large bowl, combine the plain yogurt, butter, Jamaican jerk seasoning, salt, and black pepper. Add the tempeh and toss to coat evenly. Allow marinating for 15 minutes.

In a food processor, blend the tofu with the almond meal until finely combined. Pour the mixture onto a wide plate.

Remove the tempeh from the marinade, shake off any excess liquid, and coat generously in the tofu mixture. Place on the baking sheet and grease lightly with cooking spray.

Bake in the oven for 40 to 45 minutes or until golden brown and crispy, turning once.

Remove the tempeh and serve warm with red cabbage slaw and parsnip fries.

Nutrition:

Calories:684, Total Fat:68g, Saturated Fat:12.1g, Total Carbs:13g, Dietary Fiber:4g, Sugar:1g, Protein:13g, Sodium:653mg

148. Zucchini Seitan Stacks

Preparation Time: 15 minutes

Cooking Time: 18 minutes

Servings: 4

Ingredients:

1 ½ lb seitan

3 tbsp almond flour

Salt and black pepper to taste

2 large zucchinis, cut into 2-inch slices

4 tbsp olive oil

2 tsp Italian mixed herb blend

½ cup vegetable broth

Directions:

Preheat the oven to 400 F.

Cut the seitan into strips and set aside.

In a zipper bag, add the almond flour, salt, and black pepper. Mix and add the seitan slices. Seal the bag and shake to coat the seitan with the seasoning.

Grease a baking sheet with cooking spray and arrange the zucchinis on the baking sheet. Season with salt and black pepper, and drizzle with 2 tablespoons of olive oil.

Using tongs, remove the seitan from the almond flour mixture, shake off the excess flour, and put two to three seitan strips on each zucchini.

Season with the herb blend and drizzle again with olive oil.

Cook in the oven for 8 minutes; remove the sheet and carefully pour in the vegetable broth. Bake further for 5 to 10 minutes or until the seitan cooks through.

Remove from the oven and serve warm with low carb bread.

Nutrition:

Calories:582, Total Fat:49.7g, Saturated Fat:18.4g, Total Carbs:8g, Dietary Fiber:3g, Sugar:2g, Protein:31g, Sodium:385mg

149. Curried Tofu Meatballs

Preparation Time: 5 minutes

Cooking Time: 25 minutes

Servings: 4

Ingredients:

3 lb ground tofu

1 medium yellow onion, finely chopped

2 green bell peppers, deseeded and chopped

3 garlic cloves, minced

2 tbsp melted butter

1 tsp dried parsley

2 tbsp hot sauce

Salt and ground black pepper to taste

1 tbsp red curry powder

3 tbsp olive oil

Directions:

Preheat the oven to 400 F and grease a baking sheet with cooking spray.

In a bowl, combine the tofu, onion, bell peppers, garlic, butter, parsley, hot sauce, salt, black pepper, and curry powder. With your hands, form 1-inch tofu ball from the mixture and place on the greased baking sheet.

Drizzle the olive oil over the meat and bake in the oven until the tofu ball brown on the outside and cook within, 20 to 25 minutes.

Remove the dish from the oven and plate the tofu ball.

Garnish with some scallions and serve warm on a bed of spinach salad with herbed vegan paneer cheese dressing.

Nutrition:

Calories:506, Total Fat:45.6g, Saturated Fat:18.9g, Total Carbs:11g, Dietary Fiber:1g, Sugar:1g, Protein:19g, Sodium:794mg

150. Spicy Mushroom Collard Wraps

Preparation Time: 10 minutes

Cooking Time: 16 minutes

Servings: 4

Ingredients:

2 tbsp avocado oil

1 large yellow onion, chopped

2 garlic cloves, minced

Salt and ground black pepper to taste

1 small jalapeño pepper, deseeded and finely chopped

1 ½ lb mushrooms, cut into 1-inch cubes

1 cup cauliflower rice

2 tsp hot sauce

8 collard leaves

¼ cup plain unsweetened yogurt for topping

Directions:

Heat 2 tablespoons of avocado oil in a large deep skillet; add and sauté the onion until softened, 3 minutes.

Pour in the garlic, salt, black pepper, and jalapeño pepper; cook until fragrant, 1 minute.

Mix in the mushrooms and cook both sides, 10 minutes.

Add the cauliflower rice, and hot sauce. Sauté until the cauliflower slightly softens, 2 to 3 minutes. Adjust the taste with salt and black pepper.

Lay out the collards on a clean flat surface and spoon the curried mixture onto the middle part of the leaves, about 3 tablespoons per leaf. Spoon the plain yogurt on top, wrap the leaves, and serve immediately.

Nutrition:

Calories:380, Total Fat:34.8g, Saturated Fat:19.9g, Total Carbs:10g, Dietary Fiber:5g, Sugar:5g, Protein:10g, Sodium:395mg

151. Pesto Tofu Zoodles

Preparation Time: 5minutes

Cooking Time: 12minutes

Servings size 4

Ingredients:

2 tbsp olive oil

1 medium white onion, chopped

1 garlic clove, minced

2 (14 ozblocks firm tofu, pressed and cubed

1 medium red bell pepper, deseeded and sliced

6 medium zucchinis, spiralized

Salt and black pepper to taste

¼ cup basil pesto, olive oil based

2/3 cup grated parmesan cheese

½ cup shredded mozzarella cheese

Toasted pine nuts to garnish

Directions:

Heat the olive oil in a medium pot over medium heat; sauté the onion and garlic until softened and fragrant, 3 minutes.

Add the tofu and cook until golden on all sides then pour in the bell pepper and cook until softened, 4 minutes.

Mix in the zucchinis, pour the pesto on top, and season with salt and black pepper. Cook for 3 to 4 minutes or until the zucchinis soften a little bit. Turn the heat off and carefully stir in the parmesan cheese.

Dish into four plates, share the mozzarella cheese on top, garnish with the pine nuts, and serve warm.

Nutrition:

Calories:79, Total Fat:6.2g, Saturated Fat:3.7g, Total Carbs:5g, Dietary Fiber:2g, Sugar:3g, Protein:2g, Sodium:54mg

152. Cheesy Mushroom Pie

Preparation Time: 12minutes

Cooking Time: 43minutes

Servings: 4

Ingredients:

For the piecrust:

¼ cup almond flour + extra for dusting

3 tbsp coconut flour

½ tsp salt

¼ cup butter, cold and crumbled

3 tbsp erythritol

1 ½ tsp vanilla extract

4 whole eggs

For the filling:

2 tbsp butter

1 medium yellow onion

2 garlic cloves, minced

2 cups mixed mushrooms, chopped

1 green bell pepper, deseeded and diced

1 cup green beans, cut into 3 pieces each

Salt and black pepper to taste

¼ cup coconut cream

1/3 cup vegan sour cream

½ cup almond milk

2 eggs, lightly beaten

¼ tsp nutmeg powder

1 tbsp chopped parsley

1 cup grated parmesan cheese

Directions:

For the pastry crust:

Preheat the oven to 350 F and grease a pie pan with cooking spray

In a large bowl, mix the almond flour, coconut flour, and salt.

Add the butter and mix with an electric hand mixer until crumbly. Add the erythritol and vanilla extract until mixed in. Then, pour in the eggs one after another while mixing until formed into a ball.

Flatten the dough a clean flat surface, cover in plastic wrap, and refrigerate for 1 hour.

After, lightly dust a clean flat surface with almond flour, unwrap the dough, and roll out the dough into a large rectangle, ½ - inch thickness and fit into a pie pan.

Pour some baking beans onto the pastry and bake in the oven until golden. Remove after, pour the beans, and allow cooling.

For the filling:

Meanwhile, melt the butter in a skillet and sauté the onion and garlic until softened and fragrant, 3 minutes. Add the mushrooms, bell pepper, green beans, salt and black pepper; cook for 5 minutes.

In a medium bowl, beat the coconut cream, vegan sour cream, milk, and eggs. Season with black pepper, salt, and nutmeg. Stir in the parsley and cheese.

Spread the mushroom mixture in the baked pastry and spread the cheese filling on top. Place the pie in the oven and bake for 30 to 35 minutes or until a toothpick inserted into the pie comes out clean and golden on top.

Remove, let cool for 10 minutes, slice, and serve with roasted tomato salad.

Nutrition:

Calories:120, Total Fat:9.2g, Saturated Fat:2.3g, Total Carbs:7g, Dietary Fiber:3g, Sugar:3g, Protein:5g, Sodium:17mg

153. Tofu Scallopini with Lemon

Preparation Time: 5minutes

Cooking Time: 21minutes

Servings: 4

Ingredients:

1½ lb thin cut tofu chops, boneless

Salt and ground black pepper to taste

1 tbsp avocado oil

3 tbsp butter

2 tbsp capers

1 cup vegetable broth

½ lemon, juiced + 1 lemon, sliced

2 tbsp freshly chopped parsley

Directions:

Heat the avocado oil in a large skillet over medium heat. Season the tofu chops with salt and black pepper; cook in the oil on both sides until brown and cooked through, 12 to 15 minutes. Transfer to a plate, cover with another plate, and keep warm.

Add the butter to the pan to melt and cook the capers until hot and sizzling stirring frequently to avoid burning, 3 minutes.

Pour in the vegetable broth and lemon juice, use a spatula to scrape any bits stuck to the bottom of the pan, and allow boiling until the sauce reduces by half.

Add the tofu back to the sauce, arrange the lemon slices on top, and sprinkle with half of the parsley. Allow simmering for 3 minutes.

Plate the food, garnish with the remaining parsley, and serve warm with creamy mashed cauliflower.

Nutrition:

Calories:214, Total Fat:15.6g, Saturated Fat:2.5g, Total Carbs:12g, Dietary Fiber:2g, Sugar:6g, Protein:9g, Sodium:280mg

154. Tofu Chops with Green Beans and Avocado Sauté

Preparation Time: 10minutes

Cooking Time: 22 minutes

Servings: 4

Ingredients:

For the tofu chops:

2 tbsp avocado oil

4 slices firm tofu

Salt and ground black pepper to taste

For the green beans and avocado sauté:

2 tbsp avocado oil

1 ½ cups green beans

2 large avocados, halved, pitted, and chopped

Salt and ground black pepper to taste

6 green onions, chopped

1 tbsp freshly chopped parsley

Directions:

For the tofu chops:

Heat the avocado oil in a medium skillet, season the tofu with salt and black pepper, and fry in the oil on both sides until brown, and cooked through, 12 to 15 minutes. Transfer to a plate and set aside in a warmer for serving.

For the green beans and avocado sauté:

 Heat the avocado oil in a medium skillet, add and sauté the green beans until sweating and slightly softened, 10 minutes. Mix in the avocados (don't worry if they mash up a bit), season with salt and black pepper, and the half of the green onions. Warm the avocados for 2 minutes. Turn the heat off.

Dish the sauté into serving plates, garnish with the remaining green onions and parsley, and serve with the tofu chops.

Nutrition:

Calories:503, Total Fat:41.9g, Saturated Fat:14.5g, Total Carbs:18g, Dietary Fiber:2g, Sugar:4g, Protein:19g, Sodium:314mg

155. Mushroom in Tortillas

Preparation Time: 15minutes

Cooking Time: 6hours, 64minutes

Servings: 4

Ingredients:

For the mushrooms:

2 tbsp olive oil

½ cup sliced yellow onion

2 lb mushroom

4 tbsp ras el hanout seasoning

Salt to taste

3 ½ cups vegetable broth

For the keto tortillas:

5 tbsp psyllium husk powder

1¼ cups almond flour

1 tsp salt

2 eggs, cracked into a bowl

1 cup water

2 tbsp butter, for frying

Directions:

For the mushroom:

In a large pot, heat the olive oil and sauté the onion for 3 minutes or until softened. Season the mushrooms with ras el hanout, salt, and place in the onion. Sear on each side for 3 minutes and pour the vegetable broth on top. Cover the lid, reduce the heat to low and cook for 4 to 5 hours or until the mushroom softens.

After, open the lid and shred the mushroom with two forks. Cook further over low heat for 1 hour to allow the spices to penetrate the meat strands.

Turn the heat off and using a slotted spoon, transfer the meat onto a plate. Set aside in a warmer for serving.

For the keto tortillas:

In a medium bowl, combine the psyllium husk powder, almond flour, and salt. Mix in the eggs until a thick dough forms and then the water. Separate the dough into 8 or 10 pieces.

Lay a parchment paper on a flat surface, grease with a little cooking spray, and put a dough piece on top. Cover with another parchment paper and using a rolling pin, flatten the dough into a circle. Repeat the same process for the remaining dough balls.

Melt a quarter of the butter in a large skillet over medium heat and fry the flattened dough one after another on both sides until light brown and cooked through, 40 minutes in total.

Transfer the keto tortillas to serving plates, spoon the shredded meat onto the keto tortillas and top with some leafy greens. Serve immediately.

Remove; allow cooling, and serve almond flour poppadum and coconut chutney.

Nutrition:

Calories:345, Total Fat:26.1g, Saturated Fat:15.4g, Total Carbs:11g, Dietary Fiber:5g, Sugar:5g, Protein:20g, Sodium:402mg

156. Hazelnuts and Cheese Stuffed Zucchinis

Preparation Time: 15minutes

Cooking Time: 20minutes

Servings: 4

Ingredients:

2 tbsp olive oil

1 cup cauliflower rice

¼ cup vegetable broth

1 ¼ cup diced tomatoes

1 medium red onion, chopped

¼ cup pine nuts

¼ cup hazelnuts

4 tbsp chopped cilantro

1 tbsp balsamic vinegar

1 tbsp smoked paprika

4 medium zucchinis, halved

1 cup grated parmesan cheese

Directions:

Preheat the oven to 350 F.

Pour the cauli rice and vegetable broth in a medium pot and cook over medium heat for 5 minutes or until softened. Turn the heat off, fluff the cauli rice, and allow cooling.

Scoop the flesh out of the zucchini halves using a spoon and chop the pulp. Brush the inner parts of the vegetable with olive oil.

In a bowl, mix the cauliflower rice, tomatoes, red onion, pine nuts, hazelnuts, cilantro, balsamic vinegar, paprika, zucchini pulp, salt, and black pepper.

Spoon the mixture into the zucchini halves, drizzle with more olive oil, and sprinkle the cheese on top.

Place the stuffed vegetables on a baking sheet and bake in the oven for 15 to 20 minutes or until the cheese has melted and golden.

Remove, allow cooling, and serve.

Nutrition:

Calories:197, Total Fat:15.6g, Saturated Fat:9.3g, Total Carbs:5g, Dietary Fiber:0g, Sugar:1g, Protein:9g, Sodium:1179mg

157. Tempeh Stuffed Mushrooms

Preparation Time: 5minutes

Cooking Time: 20minutes

Servings: 4

Ingredients:

2 tbsp butter

½ lb ground tempeh

Salt and ground black pepper to taste

1 tsp paprika

3 tbsp fresh chives, finely chopped

7 oz cashew cream

12 medium portabella mushrooms, stalks removed

¼ cup shredded Soy cheese

Directions:

Preheat the oven to 400 F and grease a baking sheet with cooking spray. Set aside.

Melt the butter in a medium skillet over medium heat; add the tempeh, season with salt, black pepper, and paprika. Cook until brown, 10 minutes while frequently stirring to break any lumps that form. Turn the heat off and mix in two-thirds of the chives and all the cashew cream until evenly combined.

Place the mushrooms on the baking sheet and spoon the mixture into the mushrooms. Top with the Soy cheese and bake in the oven until the mushrooms turn golden and the cheese melted, 10 minutes.

Remove the stuffed mushrooms onto serving plates, garnish with the remaining chives, and serve immediately.

Nutrition:

Calories:159, Total Fat:14.6g, Saturated Fat:7.9g, Total Carbs:3g, Dietary Fiber:0g, Sugar:0g, Protein:5g, Sodium:94mg

158. Mushroom and Vegan Bacon Lettuce Wraps

Preparation Time: 10minutes

Cooking Time: 15minutes

Servings: 4

Ingredients:

8 vegan bacon slices, chopped

2 tbsp olive oil

½ cup sliced cremini mushrooms

Salt and ground black pepper to taste

1½ lb crumbled tempeh

1 iceberg lettuce, leaves separated and washed

1 cup shredded cheddar cheese

Directions:

In a large skillet, add the bacon and cook over medium heat until brown and crispy. Transfer onto a paper-towel-lined plate and set aside.

Add the 1 tablespoon of olive oil to the skillet to heat and sauté the mushrooms. Season with salt and black pepper; allow cooking for 5 minutes or until softened.

Add the remaining oil to the skillet to heat and cook the tempeh (season with salt and black pepperuntil brown, 10 minutes, while breaking the lumps that form. Turn the heat off.

Divide the tempeh into the lettuce leaves, sprinkle with the cheddar cheese, top with the vegan bacon and mushrooms. Wrap the leaves and serve immediately with mayonnaise.

Nutrition:

Calories:447, Total Fat:43.6g, Saturated Fat:26.4g, Total Carbs:13g, Dietary Fiber:1g, Sugar:0g, Protein:10g, Sodium:1403mg

159. Mushroom in Thai Curry Sauce

Preparation Time: 15minutes

Cooking Time: 25minutes, 30seconds

Servings: 4

Ingredients:

6 tbsp butter

1 medium canon cabbage, shredded

Salt and ground black pepper to taste

1 lb mushrooms

1 celery, chopped

1 tbsp red curry powder

1 ¼ cups coconut cream

Directions:

Melt 2 tablespoons of butter in a medium skillet, add and sauté the cabbage until soft and slightly golden, and season with salt and black pepper, 5 minutes. Spoon the cabbage onto a plate and set aside.

Melt 2 tablespoons of butter in the skillet, season the mushroom with salt and black pepper, and fry in the fat until brown on the outside and cooked within, 10 minutes. Remove onto a plate and set aside.

Add the remaining butter to the skillet and once melted, sauté the celery until softened. Mix in the curry powder, heat for 30 seconds and stir in the coconut cream. Allow simmering for 5 to 10 minutes. Season with salt and black pepper.

Put the meat in the sauce and spoon some sauce over the mushroom. Turn the heat off.

Serve the mushroom and curry sauce with the buttered cabbage.

Nutrition:

Calories:310, Total Fat:24.5g, Saturated Fat:11.8g, Total Carbs:10g, Dietary Fiber:2g, Sugar:5g, Protein:16g, Sodium:136mg

160. Baked Camembert Cheese with Seitan and Pecans

Preparation Time: 8minutes

Cooking Time: 22minutes

Servings: 4

Ingredients:

9 oz whole Camembert cheese

3 tbsp olive oil

½ lb seitan chops, cut into small cubes

Salt and ground black pepper to taste

2 oz pecans

1 garlic clove, minced

1 tbsp freshly chopped parsley

Directions:

Preheat the oven to 400 F.

While the cheese is in its box, using a knife, score around the top and side of about a ¼ -inch into the cheese and take off the top layer of the skin.

Place the cheese on a baking tray and melt in the oven for 8 to 10 minutes.

Remove the cheese from the oven after.

For the topping:

Meanwhile, heat the olive oil in a medium skillet over medium heat, season the seitan with salt and black pepper, and fry in the oil until brown on all sides with a little crust, 10 to 12 minutes. Transfer to a medium mixing bowl and add the pecans, garlic, and parsley.

Spoon the mixture onto the cheese and bake in the oven for 10 minutes or until the cheese softens and nuts toasts.

Serve warm with low carb bread or steamed asparagus.

Nutrition:

Calories:266, Total Fat:24.9g, Saturated Fat:4.7g, Total Carbs:6g, Dietary Fiber:1g, Sugar:2g, Protein:7g, Sodium:232mg

161. Cheesy Tempeh Burrito Bowl

Preparation Time: 10minutes

Cooking Time: 15minutes

Servings: 4

Ingredients:

1 tbsp butter

1 lb ground tempeh

½ cup vegetable broth

4 tbsp taco seasoning

Salt and ground black pepper to taste

½ cup sharp cheddar cheese, shredded

½ cup sour cream

¼ cup sliced black olives

1 avocado, cubed

¼ cup tomatoes, diced

1 green onion, sliced

1 tbsp fresh cilantro, chopped

Directions:

Melt the butter in a large skillet over medium heat. Add and cook the tempeh until brown while breaking any lumps that form, 10 minutes.

Mix in the vegetable broth, taco seasoning, salt, and black pepper; cook until most of the liquid has evaporated, 5 minutes.

Mix in half of the cheddar cheese and allow melting. Turn the heat off.

Spoon the dish into a large serving bowl and top with the olives, avocado, tomatoes, green onion, and cilantro.

Serve warm with low carb tortillas.

Nutrition:

Calories:530, Total Fat:57.5g, Saturated Fat:8.9g, Total Carbs:3g, Dietary Fiber:1g, Sugar:1g, Protein:3g, Sodium:8mg

162. Tofu Casserole with Cottage Cheese

Preparation Time: 5 minutes

Cooking Time: 5 minutes

Servings: 4

Ingredients:

2 tbsp avocado oil

1½ lb crumbled tofu

Salt and black pepper to taste

¼ cup sliced Kalamata olives

½ cup cottage cheese, crumbled

2 garlic cloves, minced

½ cup unsweetened marinara sauce

1 ¼ cups heavy cream

Directions:

Preheat the oven to 400 F and lightly grease a casserole dish with cooking spray. Set aside.

Heat the avocado oil in a deep, medium skillet over medium heat, add the tofu, season with salt and black pepper, and cook until brown, 10 minutes. Stir frequently.

Transfer and spread the tofu in the bottom of the casserole dish. Scatter the olives, cottage cheese, and garlic on top.

In a medium bowl, mix the marinara sauce and heavy cream, and pour the mixture all over the other Ingredients.

Bake in the oven until the top is bubbly and lightly brown, 20 to 30 minutes.

Remove after and dish into serving plates.

Serve warm with a leafy green salad.

Nutrition:

Calories:511, Total Fat:46.4g, Saturated Fat:7.5g, Total Carbs:13g, Dietary Fiber:4g, Sugar:5g, Protein:16g, Sodium:153mg

163. Egg Roll and Tofu Bowl

Preparation Time: 15minutes

Cooking Time: 15minutes

Servings: 4

Ingredients:

2 tbsp sesame oil

2 large eggs

2 tbsp minced garlic

½ tsp ginger puree

1 medium white onion, diced

1 lb ground tofu

Salt and ground black pepper to taste

1 habanero pepper, chopped

1 small green cabbage, shredded

5 scallions, chopped

3 tbsp coconut aminos

1 tbsp white vinegar

2 tbsp sesame seeds

Directions:

Heat 1 tablespoon of sesame oil in a medium skillet over medium heat and scramble the eggs until set, 1 minute. Transfer to a plate and set aside.

Heat the remaining sesame oil in the same skillet and sauté the garlic, ginger, and onion in the same skillet until softened and fragrant, 4 minutes.

Add the ground tofu, season with salt, black pepper, and habanero pepper. Cook until the tofu turns brown, 10 minutes.

Mix in the cabbage, scallions, coconut aminos, and vinegar and cook until the cabbage is tender. Stir in the eggs and adjust the taste with salt and black pepper.

Dish the food, garnish with the sesame seeds, and serve with low carb tortillas.

Nutrition:

Calories:319, Total Fat:23.1g, Saturated Fat:13.4g, Total Carbs:7g, Dietary Fiber:2g, Sugar:4g, Protein:21g, Sodium:1060mg

164. Tempeh Chops with Caramelized Onions and Brie Cheese

Preparation Time: 10minutes

Cooking Time: 35minutes

Servings: 4

Ingredients:

3 tbsp olive oil

2 large red onions, sliced

2 tbsp balsamic vinegar

1 tsp sugar-free maple syrup

Salt and ground black pepper to taste

4 mushroom chops

4 slices brie cheese

2 tbsp freshly chopped mint leaves

Directions:

Heat 1 tablespoon of olive oil in a medium skillet over medium heat until starting to smoke. Reduce the heat to low and sauté the onions until golden brown. Pour in the vinegar, maple syrup, and salt. Cook with frequent stirring to prevent burning until the onions caramelize, 20 minutes. Transfer to a plate and set aside.

Heat the remaining olive oil in the same skillet, season the mushroom with salt and black pepper, and cook in the oil until cooked and brown on the outside, 10 to 12 minutes.

Put a brie slice on each meat and top with the caramelized onions. Allow the cheese to melt for 2 to 3 minutes.

Carefully spoon the meat with topping onto serving plates and garnish with the mint leaves.

Serve immediately with buttered radishes.

Nutrition:

Calories:680, Total Fat:71.8g, Saturated Fat:20.9g, Total Carbs:10g, Dietary Fiber:7g, Sugar:2g, Protein:3g, Sodium:525mg

165. Coconut Mushroom Dumplings

Preparation Time: 10minutes

Cooking Time: 12minutes

Servings: 4

Ingredients:

1 lb ground mushroom

2 scallions, chopped

1 small cucumber, deseeded and grated

4 garlic cloves, minced

1 tsp freshly pureed ginger

1 tsp red chili flakes

2 tbsp tamari sauce

2 tbsp sesame oil

3 tbsp coconut oil, for frying

Directions:

In a medium bowl, combine the mushroom, scallions, cucumber, garlic, ginger, red chili flakes, tamari sauce, and sesame oil. Using your hands, form 1-inch oval shapes out of the mixture and place on a plate.

Heat the coconut oil in a medium skillet over medium heat; fry the dumplings until brown on both sides and cooked, 12 minutes.

Transfer to a paper towel-lined plate to drain grease and serve with creamy spinach puree.

Nutrition:

Calories:439, Total Fat:31.9g, Saturated Fat:12.2g, Total Carbs:9g, Dietary Fiber:4g, Sugar:1g, Protein:36g, Sodium:574mg

166. Brown Rice Stir Fry with Vegetables

Cooking time: 25 minutes

Servings: 4

Ingredients

1 handful fresh parsley, chopped

1/2 zucchini, chopped

2 tablespoons olive oil

2 tablespoons soy sauce

1/2 bell pepper, chopped

1/2 cup brown rice, uncooked

4 garlic cloves, minced

1 cup red cabbage, chopped

1/8 teaspoon cayenne powder

1/2 broccoli head, chopped

Sesame seeds, for garnish

Directions:

Cook the brown rice as per the package instructions.

Bring water to a boil in a frying pan and then add veggies and make sure they are fully covered with water. Cook for 1-2 minutes on high heat, and then drain the water and set aside.

Add oil to the wok pan and heat over high heat and then add garlic along with parsley and cayenne powder. Cook for a minute stirring frequently and then add the drained veggies, tamari and the cooked rice.

Cook for 1-2 minutes and then garnish with sesame seeds if desired. Serve and enjoy!

167. Grilled Veggie Skewers

Cooking time: 15 minutes

Servings: 4-6

Ingredients

1 red onion, peeled, chopped

2 tablespoons avocado oil

2 portobello mushrooms, chopped

1 sweet potato, chopped

2 bell peppers, chopped

6 baby red potatoes, quartered

Salt and black pepper, to taste

4 ears corn

Directions:

Preheat the oven to 375F and add the sweet potato to a cooking pot along with the quartered potatoes and water. Bring to a boil and cook until lightly tender for about 10 minutes. When done, drain the water and let cool a bit.

Thread the vegetables onto skewers, and then brush them evenly with oil. When done, season the vegetables generously with salt and pepper on each side.

Cook the vegetables for about 10-15 minutes until tender and cooked through. Flip halfway. Place the corn directly on the vegetables to cook together.

When done, serve and enjoy with the desired sauce.

168. Eggplant Teriyaki Bowls

Cooking time: 45 minutes

Servings: 4

INGREDIENTS

1 carrot, shredded

1 chucky eggplant

¼ cup edamame beans, frozen

1 lime, ½ sliced, ½ juiced

2 spring onions , chopped

1 ½ tablespoons vegetable oil

1 handful radishes, sliced

1 tablespoon caster sugar

1 garlic clove, crushed

½ cup jasmine rice

2 tablespoons sesame seeds, toasted

1 small ginger, grated

2 tablespoons soy sauce

DIRECTIONS:

Add 2 cups of water to a cooking pan, add rice and salt to taste. Bring to a boil, cook for a minute, and then close the lid. Reduce the heat to low and cook for 10 minutes until cooked through. Turn off the heat and steam for additional 10 minutes.

Add a tablespoon of oil to a bowl and toss the eggplant in it. Preheat the wok pan, add the eggplant and cook for 5 minutes, stirring often, until lightly softened and charred. Add the carrots to the wok along with garlic, ginger and spring onions, and then fry for 2-3 minutes.

In a small bowl, whisk the sugar along with soy sauce and a cup of water and then add into the wok. Simmer until the eggplant is very soft, for about 10-15 minutes.

Add water to the pan and bring to a boil and then add the frozen edamame beans, remove the beans, drain and rinse them well under running water. Add the radishes to a bowl, drain the beans again and then add them to the radishes. Squeeze lime juice on top and toss well until combined.

Serve the rice in the bowls and then scoop the eggplant and sauce on top along with the beans and radishes. Sprinkle with sesame seeds and garnish with the lime slices. Enjoy

169. Quinoa and Black Bean Chilli

Cooking time: 45 minutes

Servings: 8

Ingredients

3 cups vegetable stock

1 onion, chopped

1 cup quinoa, rinsed, drained

1 red chilli, chopped

2 teaspoons ground cumin

1 lb. tomatoes, chopped

olive oil spray

1 teaspoon smoked paprika

1 small avocado, sliced

½ teaspoon chilli powder

2 garlic cloves, crushed

1 lb. black beans, rinsed, drained

Coriander leaves, to serve

Directions:

Generously grease the cooking pan with oil and place over medium heat and then add the onion, red chili and garlic. Fry the ingredients until soft, and then add spices and stir.

Add the vegetable stock into the pan along with quinoa, black beans and tomatoes, and then adjust the seasonings if needed.

Close the lid and simmer until quinoa is tender, for about 30 minutes.

When done, garnish with coriander leaves and top with the avocado slices. Serve and enjoy!

170. Mac and Cheese

Cooking Time: 20 minutes

Servings: 4

Ingredients

8 oz. whole-grain macaroni elbows, cooked

1 head of broccoli, florets

1 ½ tablespoons avocado oil

1 onion, chopped

1 cup potato, peeled and grated

3 cloves garlic, minced

½ teaspoon garlic powder

½ teaspoon onion powder

½ teaspoon dry mustard powder

1 small pinch red pepper flakes

⅔ cup raw cashews

1 cup water, or more if needed

¼ cup nutritional yeast

3 teaspoons apple cider vinegar

salt

Directions:

Place a large pot over medium heat. Add salt and water and bring to a boil.

Add broccoli and cook for 5 minutes. Once done, drain excess liquid and set aside in a large mixing bowl.

Place a large skillet over medium heat. Add oil.

Add onion, salt and cook for about 5 minutes.

Add potatoes, garlic, garlic powder, onion powder, mustard powder, salt, red pepper flakes and cook for 60 seconds.

Add cashews, water, bring mixture to a simmer, reduce the heat and let it cook until potatoes are tender. Remove from the heat.

Pour the mixture into a food processor, add nutritional yeast, vinegar and pulse until the mixture is smooth, adding water if necessary.

Serve cooked pasta in bowls, topped with the blended mixture.

171. Butternut Squash Linguine with Fried Sage

Cooking Time: 25 minutes

Servings: 4

Ingredients

3 cups butternut squash, peeled, seeded, and chopped

2 cups vegetable broth

12 oz. whole grain fettucine, cooked, 1 cup cooking liquid saved

1 onion, chopped

2 garlic cloves, pressed

2 tablespoons olive oil

1 tablespoon fresh sage, chopped

⅛ teaspoon red pepper flakes

salt and pepper

Directions:

Place a large pan over medium heat. Add oil.

Add sage and cook it until crispy. Season with salt and set aside.

Return the same pan to medium heat, add butternut, onion, garlic, red pepper flakes, salt and pepper. Cook for about 10 minutes.

Add broth and bring to a boil, then reduce the heat and let it cook for 20 minutes.

Place a pot of salty water over medium heat.

Cool the squash mixture and blend the mixture until smooth with a mixer.

Add pasta, ¼ cup reserved pasta liquid to the pan, return pan to medium heat and cook for 3 minutes.

172. Paella

Cooking Time: 1 hour

Servings: 6

Ingredients

15 oz. diced tomatoes, drained

2 cups short-grain brown rice

1 ½ cups cooked chickpeas

3 cups vegetable broth

⅓ cup dry white wine

1 14 oz. artichokes, drained and chopped

½ cup Kalamata olives, pitted and halved

¼ cup parsley, chopped

½ cup peas

3 tablespoons extra-virgin olive oil, divided

1 onion, chopped

6 garlic cloves, pressed or minced

2 teaspoons smoked paprika

½ teaspoon saffron threads, crumbled

2 bell peppers, stemmed, seeded and sliced

2 tablespoons lemon juice

salt and pepper

Directions:

Preheat the oven to 350F.

Place a large skillet over medium heat and add 2 tablespoons oil.

Add onion, salt and cook for 5 minutes.

Add garlic, paprika and cook for ½ a minute.

Add tomatoes and stir well. Cook until the mixture starts to thicken.

Add rice and cook for 1 minute while stirring.

Add chickpeas, broth, wine, saffron and salt to taste. Increase the heat and bring the mixture to a boil. Remove from the heat.

Cover and immediately transfer to an oven on lower rack. Bake for 1 hour.

Prepare a baking sheet by lining it with parchment paper. Combine artichokes, peppers, olives, 1 tablespoon olive oil, salt and pepper. Mix well and roast vegetables on the upper rack in the oven for 45 minutes.

Add parsley and lemon juice to the baking pan and mix well.

Sprinkle the roasted vegetables and peas on the baked rice.

173. Spicy Thai Peanut Sauce Over Roasted Sweet Potatoes and Rice

Cooking Time: 1 hour 30 minutes

Servings: 4

Ingredients

For the spicy Thai peanut sauce:

½ cup creamy peanut butter

¼ cup reduced-sodium tamari

3 tablespoons apple cider vinegar

2 tablespoons honey or maple syrup

1 teaspoon grated fresh ginger

2 cloves garlic, pressed

¼ teaspoon red pepper flakes

2 tablespoons water

For the roasted vegetables:

2 sweet potatoes, peeled and sliced

1 bell pepper, cored, deseeded, and sliced

about 2 tablespoons coconut oil (or olive oil)

¼ teaspoon cumin powder

salt

For the rice and garnishes:

1 ¼ cup jasmine brown rice

2 green onions, sliced

a handful of cilantro, torn

a handful of peanuts, crushed

Directions:

Place a pot of water on medium heat and bring it to a boil.

Preheat the oven to 425F.

On a rimmed baking sheet, mix sweet potato, 1 tablespoon coconut oil, cumin and salt. Roast in the middle rack for about 35 minutes.

On another baking sheet, mix bell pepper with 1 teaspoon coconut oil, salt and mix well, Roast on the top rack for about 20 minutes until tender.

When water is boiling in the pot add rice and mix well. Cook for about 30 minutes and drain excess liquid. Once done, cover and let it sit for 10 minutes, fluff it after.

Mix sauce ingredients in a small bowl and set aside.

Divide rice, roasted vegetables in bowls and top with sauce, green onions, cilantro and peanuts before serving.

174. Butternut Squash Chipotle Chili With Avocado

Cooking Time: 20 minutes

Servings: 4

Ingredients

3 cups black beans, cooked

14 oz. can diced tomatoes, including the liquid

2 cups vegetable broth

1 onion, chopped

2 bell peppers, chopped

1 small butternut squash, cubed

4 garlic cloves, minced

2 tablespoons olive oil

1 tablespoon chili powder

½ tablespoon chopped chipotle pepper in adobo

1 teaspoon ground cumin

¼ teaspoon ground cinnamon

1 bay leaf

2 avocados, diced

3 corn tortillas for crispy tortilla strips

salt

Directions:

Place a stockpot over medium heat. Add oil.

Add and cook onion, bell peppers and butternut squash for about 5 minutes.

Reduce the heat, add garlic, chili powder, ½ tablespoon chopped chipotle peppers, cumin and cinnamon. Cook for ½ a minute.

Add bay leaves, black beans, tomatoes and their juices and broth. Mix well. Cook for about 1 hour. Remove bay leaf when done cooking.

Slice corn tortillas into thin little strips.

Place a pan over medium heat and add olive oil. Add tortilla strips and season with salt. Cook until crispy for about 7 minutes. Remove from the heat and place in a bowl covered with paper towel to drain excess oil.

Serve chili in bowls, topped with crispy tortilla chips and avocado.

175. Chickpea Biryani

Cooking Time: 40 minutes

Servings: 6

Ingredients

4 cups veggie stock

2 cups basmati rice, rinsed

1 can chickpeas, drained, rinsed

½ cup raisins

1 large onion, thinly sliced

2 cups thinly sliced veggies (bell pepper, zucchini and carrots)

3 garlic cloves, chopped

1 tablespoon ginger, chopped

1 tablespoon cumin

1 tablespoon coriander

1 teaspoon chili powder

1 teaspoon cinnamon

½ teaspoon cardamom

½ teaspoon turmeric

2 tablespoons olive oil

1 bay leaf

salt

Directions:

Place a large skillet over medium high heat. Add oil.

Sauté onions for about 5 minutes.

Reduce the heat to medium, add vegetables, garlic and ginger. Cook for 5 minutes. Scoop 1 cup of this mixture and set aside.

Add spices, bay leaf and rice. Stir for about 1 minute.

Add stock and salt to taste.

Add chickpeas, raisins and 1 cup of vegetables. Bring the mixture to a simmer over high heat.

Lower the heat, cover tightly and let it simmer for ½ an hour. Remove from the heat when rice is done.

176. Chinese Eggplant

Cooking Time: 45 minutes

Servings: 4

Ingredients

1 ½ lbs. eggplants, chopped

2 cups water

2 tablespoons cornstarch

4 tablespoons peanut oil

4 cloves garlic, chopped

2 teaspoons ginger, minced

10 dried red chilies

salt

For the Szechuan sauce:

1 teaspoon Szechuan peppercorns

¼ cup soy sauce

1 tablespoon garlic chili paste

1 tablespoon sesame oil

1 tablespoon rice vinegar

1 tablespoon Chinese cooking wine

3 tablespoons coconut sugar

½ teaspoon five spice

Directions:

Place chopped eggplants in a shallow bowl. Add water and 2 teaspoons salt. Stir cover and let it sit for about 15 minutes.

Meanwhile place a small pan over medium heat. Toast the Szechuan peppercorns for about 2 minutes and crush them.

Add crushed peppercorns to a medium bowl, add soy, chili paste, sesame oil, rice vinegar, Chinese cooking vinegar, coconut sugar and five spice.

Drain excess liquid from the eggplants and toss in the corn starch.

Place a large skillet over medium heat, add eggplants and cook them until golden. Set aside.

Add 1 tablespoon of oil in the skillet placed over medium heat. Cook garlic and ginger for 2 minutes.

Add dried chilies and cook for 1 minute. Add the Szechuan sauce and bring the mixture to a simmer in 20 seconds.

Add back eggplants and cook for about 60 seconds.

177. Black Pepper Tofu with Bok Choy

Cooking Time: 30 minutes

Servings: 2

Ingredients

12 oz. firm tofu, cubed

1/3 cup corn starch for dredging

2 tablespoons coconut oil

1 teaspoon fresh cracked peppercorns

1 shallot, sliced

4 cloves garlic, chopped

6 oz. baby bok choy, sliced to 4 slices

For the black pepper sauce:

2 tablespoons soy sauce

2 tablespoons Chinese cooking wine

2 tablespoons water

1 teaspoon brown sugar

½ teaspoon fresh cracked peppercorns

1 teaspoon chili paste

Directions:

In a small bowl, combine wok sauce ingredients and mix well until sugar dissolves. Set aside.

Place cornstarch in a shallow bowl and dredge tofu in the cornstarch. Set aside.

Place a large skillet over medium heat. Heat 1 tablespoon coconut oil.

Add peppercorns and toast for about 1 minute.

Add tofu and cook on all sides for about 6 minutes. Set tofu aside.

Add the remaining coconut oil. Add shallots, garlic and bok choy. Cook for 8 minutes.

Add back the tofu and cook for less than a minute.

178. Spaghetti Alla Puttanesca

Cooking Time: 30 minutes

Servings: 4

Ingredients

For the Puttanesca sauce:

28 oz. can chunky tomato sauce

⅓ cup chopped Kalamata olives

⅓ cup capers

1 tablespoon Kalamata olive brine

1 tablespoon caper brine

3 cloves garlic, minced

¼ teaspoon red pepper flakes

1 tablespoon olive oil

½ cup parsley leaves, chopped and divided

salt and pepper

For the pasta:

8 oz. whole grain spaghetti

6 oz. zucchini noodles

Directions:

Place a medium skillet over medium heat.

Add tomato sauce, olives, capers, olive brine, caper brine, garlic and red pepper flakes. Bring the mixture to a boil, reduce the heat and let it simmer for 20 minutes. Remove from the heat and set aside.

Place a pot over medium heat. Add water, salt, spaghetti and cook as directed on package. When done, drain excess water.

Pour the sauce over pasta and mix well.

Add zucchini noodles before serving.

179. Thai Red Curry

Cooking Time: 40 minutes

Servings: 4

Ingredients

1 ¼ cups brown jasmine rice, rinsed

1 tablespoon coconut oil

1 cup onion, chopped

1 tablespoon fresh ginger, ginger

2 cloves garlic, minced

1 red bell pepper, sliced

1 yellow bell pepper, sliced

3 carrots, peeled and sliced

2 tablespoons Thai red curry paste

1 14 oz. can coconut milk

½ cup water

1 ½ cups packed kale, chopped

1 ½ teaspoons coconut sugar

1 tablespoon tamari

2 teaspoons fresh lime juice

Directions:

Place a large pot over medium heat and add water. Bring it to a boil.

Add rice, salt and cook for 30 minutes. Remove from the heat, cover and let it sit for 10 minutes.

Place a large pan over medium heat. Add oil.

Cook onion and salt for about 5 minutes.

Add garlic, ginger and cook for about ½ a minute.

Add bell peppers, carrots and cook for about 5 minutes.

Add curry paste and cook for additional 2 minutes.

Add coconut milk, water, kale, sugar, tamari and lime juice. Remove from the heat.

180. Thai Green Curry with Spring Vegetables

Cooking Time: 45 minutes

Servings:4

Ingredients

1 cup brown basmati rice, rinsed

2 teaspoons coconut oil

1 onion, diced

1 tablespoon fresh ginger, chopped

2 cloves garlic, chopped

2 cups asparagus, sliced

1 cup carrots, peeled and sliced

2 tablespoons Thai green curry paste

14 oz. full-fat coconut milk (I used full-fat coconut milk for a richer curry)

½ cup water

1 ½ teaspoons coconut sugar

2 cups packed baby spinach, chopped

1 ½ teaspoons fresh lime juice

1 ½ teaspoons tamari

salt

Directions:

Place a pot over medium heat. Add water and bring it to a boil.

Add rice, salt to taste and cook for 30 minutes. When done, cover the rice and set aside for more than 10 minutes.

Place a large skillet over medium heat. Add oil.

Cook onion, garlic, ginger and a pinch of salt.

Add asparagus, carrots and cook for 3 minutes.

Add curry paste and cook for additional 2 minutes.

Add coconut milk, ½ cup water, sugar and bring this mixture to a simmer. Reduce the heat and let it cook for 10 minutes until vegetables are tender.

Add spinach and let it cook for ½ a minute. Remove from the heat and season with rice vinegar and tamari.

181. Tamarind Potato Curry

Cooking Time: 1 hour

Servings: 4

Ingredients

26.5 oz. potatoes, peeled and cubed

1 onion

1 garlic clove

1-inch ginger, chopped

1 green chilli, chopped

oil for frying

1 teaspoon cumin seeds

½ teaspoon fennel seeds

1 teaspoon ground coriander

1 teaspoon chilli powder

14 oz. plum tomatoes

2 teaspoon brown sugar

2 tablespoons tamarind paste

1 handful coriander leaves

rice or naan bread, to serve

Directions:

Place a pot of water over medium heat. Add salt and potatoes. Bring to a boil.

Place onion, garlic, ginger, chili, and 2 tablespoons water in a food processor. Pulse until smooth.

Place a pan over medium heat. Add oil.

Toast cumin and fennel seeds until they pop.

Add spices, puree and cook for 5 minutes.

Add tomatoes, sugar, tamarind and let it simmer for 10 minutes.

Add potatoes and some water. Cover and let it cook until tender.

Serve with rice or naan bread.

182. West African Stew with Sweet Potato and Greens

Cooking Time: 1 hour

Servings: 4

Ingredients

1/5 cup crunchy peanut butter

1/3 cup coconut cream

3 cups vegetable stock

21 oz. sweet potatoes, cubed

2 cups okra, halved

1 cup loosely packed kale, chopped

2 onions, 1 roughly chopped and 1 diced

1-inch ginger, chopped

3 garlic cloves

1 scotch bonnet chilli

4 tablespoons tomato purée

sunflower oil

2 teaspoons coriander seeds, toasted and crushed

2 teaspoons ground cumin

salt

Directions:

Combine roughly chopped onion, ginger, garlic, scotch bonnet, tomato puree and peanut butter in a blender. Blend for 1 minute until paste forms.

Place a cast iron pan over medium heat. Add 2 tablespoons sunflower oil.

Add diced onions and cook for 5 minutes. Season with salt.

Add spices, peanut sauce and cook for 5 minutes.

Add coconut cream, stock and bring it to a simmer for about 10 minutes.

Add cubed sweet potatoes, cover and cook for about 15 minutes.

Add okra, kale and cook for 10 additional minutes.

Remove from heat before serving.

183. Kale Slaw

Cooking Time: 15 minutes

Servings: 4

Ingredients

1 small bunch kale, chopped

½ small head cabbage, shredded

¼ onion, thinly sliced

¼ cup tender herbs (cilantro, basil, parsley, chives)

¼ cup olive oil

4 tablespoons lemon juice

2 garlic cloves, minced

salt, pepper and chili flakes

Directions:

Combine kale, cabbage, herbs and onions in a large bowl.

Add olive oil, lemon juice, minced garlic, salt, pepper and mix well.

Add chili flakes, toss well before serving.

184. Salisbury Steak and Mushroom Gravy

Preparation Time: 30 Minutes

Servings: 4

Ingredients:

4 palm-sized pieces beef seitan

1 1/2 tablespoons vegan chicken-flavored bouillon

8 ounces mushrooms, chopped

1/2 teaspoon garlic powder

1/2 teaspoon basil

1 bay leaf

1/8 teaspoon celery salt

1/8 teaspoon seasoned salt

1/4 teaspoon pepper

1 cup water

1 cup nondairy milk

2 tablespoons olive oil

1/2 cup plus 3 tablespoons flour

Directions:

Make a coating for the seitan by mixing the garlic powder, celery salt, ½ cup flour, basil, seasoned salt, and pepper in a bowl. Make sure seitan is wet before coating it with the flour mixture.

Heat the oil in the instant pot on the sauté setting. Brown the seitan steaks on each side, then set aside.

Add the water, mushrooms, bay leaf, and bouillon to the instant pot, then place the seitan on top. Seal the lid and cook on high 4 minutes, before letting the pressure release naturally.

Remove the lid and discard the bay leaf. Return to the sauté setting.

Remove the steaks, then stir in the nondairy milk. Add the flour to thicken the gravy, then add the steaks. Simmer for 10 minutes. Add additional flour if needed.

Serve with a side of mashed potatoes smothered in your mushroom gravy.

185. Savory Spinach and Mushroom Crepes

Preparation Time: 60 Minutes

Servings: 4

Ingredients:

For the crepes:

1 ¾ cup rolled oats

1 tsp pink Himalayan salt

1 ½ cup soy milk

2 tbsp olive oil

1 tbsp almond butter

½ tsp nutmeg

2 tbsp egg replacement

For the filling:

1 lb button mushrooms

10 oz fresh spinach, finely chopped

4 oz crumbled tofu

1 tbsp chia seeds

1 tbsp fresh rosemary, finely chopped

1 garlic clove, crushed

2 tbsp olive oil

Directions:

First, prepare the crepes. Combine all dry ingredients in a large bowl. Add milk, butter, nutmeg, olive oil, and egg replacement. Mix well with a hand mixer on high speed. Transfer to a food processor and process until completely smooth.

Grease a large non-stick pancake pan with some oil. Pour 1 cup of the mixture into the pan and cook for one minute on each side.

Plug in your instant pot and press the 'Sauté' button. Grease the stainless steel insert with some oil and add mushrooms. Cook for 5 minutes, stirring constantly.

Now add spinach, tofu, rosemary, and garlic. Continue to cook for another 5 minutes.

Remove the mixture from the pot and stir in chia seeds. Let it sit for 10 minutes.

Meanwhile, grease a small baking pan with some oil and line with parchment paper.

Divide the mushroom mixture between crepes and roll up. Gently transfer to a prepared baking pan.

Wrap the pan with aluminum foil and set aside.

Pour 1 cup of water in your instant pot and set the steam rack. Put the pan on top and seal the lid. Press the 'Manual' button and set the timer for 10 minutes.

When done, release the pressure naturally, and open the lid.

Optionally, sprinkle with some dried oregano before serving.

186. Stuffed Sweet Onions

Preparation Time: 45 Minutes

Servings: 5

Ingredients:

10 medium-sized sweet onions

1 lb portobello mushrooms, chopped

1 medium-sized eggplant, finely chopped

3 tbsp olive oil

1 tbsp dried mint

1 tsp cayenne pepper

½ tsp cumin powder

1 tsp salt

½ cup tomato paste

¼ cup fresh parsley, finely chopped

Directions:

Cut a ¼-inch slice from top of each onion and trim a small amount from the bottom end. This will make the onions stand upright. Place onions in a microwave-safe dish and add about 1 cup of water. Cover with a tight lid and microwave on High 2-3 minutes. Remove onions from a dish and cool slightly. Now carefully remove inner layers of onions with a sharp knife, leaving about ¼-inch onion shell.

In a large bowl, combine chopped mushrooms, eggplant, olive oil, mint, cayenne pepper, cumin powder, salt, and tomato paste. Use 1 tablespoon of the mixture to fill the onions.

Grease the bottom of the stainless steel insert with some oil and gently place onions. Add 2 cups of water or vegetable stock and seal the lid. Press the 'Manual' button and set the timer for 15 minutes.

When done, release the pressure naturally and open the lid. Sprinkle with parsley before serving.

187. Eggplant Casserole

 Preparation Time: 50 Minutes

Servings: 4

Ingredients:

1 large eggplant, sliced

7 oz button mushrooms

2 large onions, finely chopped

2 large tomatoes, sliced

7 oz cherry tomatoes, sliced

½ cup almond butter

¼ cup soaked cashews

2 tbsp egg replacement

¼ cup olive oil

1 tsp salt

½ tsp freshly ground black pepper

Directions:

Grease a round baking pan with two tablespoons of olive oil and set aside.

Plug in your instant pot and grease the stainless steel insert with the remaining oil. Press the 'Sauté' button and add onions. Stir-fry until translucent. Now add mushrooms, salt, and pepper. Continue to cook for 3-4 minutes, stirring constantly.

Finally, add almond butter and cook until melted.

Remove the mixture from your pot and transfer to a medium-sized bowl. Add tomatoes, cherry tomatoes, soaked cashews, and egg replacement. Mix well.

Spread half of the eggplant slices over the prepared pan and top with the tomato mixture. Finish with the remaining eggplant and wrap tightly with aluminum foil.

Pour in 2 cups of water in your instant pot and set the steam rack. Put the pan on top and seal the lid. Set the steam release handle and press the 'Manual' button.

Set the timer for 25 minutes.

When done, perform a quick release and open the lid. Remove the pan and chill for a while before serving.

188. Corn Chowder

Preparation Time: 20 MINS| Serves 4

Ingredients:

2 Tablespoons Vegan Butter

4 Scallions, chopped, use green tops and white bulbs and set aside separately

1 Sweet Red Bell Pepper, diced

2 Celery Stalks, diced

4 Cups Vegetable Broth

1 pound Red or New Potatoes, peeled and diced

4 Cups Corn Kernels, fresh from the cob is best, but frozen is okay

1 Bay Leaf

2 Teaspoons Sea Salt

2 Cups Unsweetened Plain Almond Milk

1/4 Teaspoon Black Pepper

Directions:

On saute mode, add butter until melted.

Add the white bulbs of the scallions, red pepper, and celery. Cook until soft.

Add broth, potatoes, corn, and bay leaf.

Season with a pinch of salt.

Put instant pot on manual mode on high. Seal the lid and set to 10 minutes.

When done cooking, release the pressure and open when steam has evaporated.

Add almond milk and pepper. Stir.

Put instant pot in saute mode and allow to boil for 2 minutes to thicken slightly.

Remove the bay leaf and stir in the green tops of the scallions.

Enjoy!

189. Lemony Roasted Vegetable Risotto

Preparation Time: 30 MINS| Serves 4

Ingredients:

3 1/2 Cups Butternut Squash, peeled, cubed

1/1/2 Cups Zucchini, diced

1 large Carrot, peeled, chopped

2 Tablespoons Olive Oil

Sea Salt + Pepper to taste

1 Onion, diced

2 Garlic Cloves, minced

6 Cups Vegetable Broth

1 Tablespoon Vegan Butter

2 Cups Arborio Rice

1/2 Cup Baby Spinach

1 Teaspoon Lemon Zest

2 Tablespoons lemon juice, more to taste

Directions:

Preheat oven to 400 degrees F. Line a baking tray with parchment paper. Add butternut squash, zucchini, and carrot to the tray. Coat with 1 teaspoon of olive oil, salt, and pepper, toss well.

Roast in the oven for 15-20 minutes or until squash is soft when poked with a fork. When done, remove from oven and set aside.

Press saute mode on instant pot. Add remaining olive oil, and when hot, cook onions and garlic for 2-3 minutes or until onions become semitransparent.

Add rice and stir for 1-2 minutes to coat.

Add broth, and vegan butter. Stir to combine.

Turn the instant pot off. Cover and seal. Press manual button and adjust the time to 7 minutes.

When done cooking, release the pressure and stir well.

Return to saute mode, add spinach and roasted vegetables.

Stir until spinach has wilted. Taste and add salt and pepper as needed.

Top with lemon juice and zest.

Best when served fresh and warm.

Enjoy!

190.   Thai Coconut Peanut Tofu

Preparation Time: 26 MIN| Serves 4

Ingredients:

1 Cup Creamy Natural Peanut Butter

1 Can (about 1 1/2 CupsLight Coconut Milk

1/2 Cup Vegetable Broth

2 Teaspoons Curry Powder

2 Tablespoons Coconut Sugar

2 Teaspoons Ground Cumin Powder

1/4 Teaspoon Sea Salt, add more to taste

1-2 Tablespoons Coconut Oil (or Olive or Sesame Oil

1 Bunch Green Onions, sliced (reserve half for garnish

2 Tablespoons minced Fresh Ginger

1 Cup Carrots, shredded

1/4 Cup Roasted Cashews, salted or unsalted

1 Pinch Cayenne Pepper

2 Tablespoons Tamari (or Soy Sauce

3 Teaspoons Rice Vinegar

1 Package(200 GramsExtra-Firm Tofu, cubed

1 Lemon, juiced

Directions:

In a bowl, mix peanut butter, coconut milk, broth, curry powder, coconut sugar, cumin, and sea salt. Make sure ingredients are mixed completely. Set aside.

Press saute mode on instant pot. When it is hot, add the coconut oil, half of the green onions, ginger, and garlic.

Add a pinch of salt and saute for 2-3 minutes, stirring frequently.

Add the carrots, cashews, cayenne, and saute for 2 minutes more.

Add the peanut butter mixture into the pot and stir well.

Then add tamari or soy sauce and rice vinegar. Stir to combine.

Lastly, add tofu to the pot and mix.

Cover and turn off saute mode. Press the manual button, change pressure to high and let cook for 2 minutes.

Quick release when 2 minutes are done.

Return to saute mode and let simmer to let tofu infuse with flavor. Add more broth if too thick.

Add lemon juice and serve over rice, quinoa, or steamed vegetables.

Garnish with the rest of the green onions and enjoy!

191. Vegan Butter Curry Tofu

Preparation Time: 77 MINS| Servings: 4-5

Ingredients:

1 1/2 Cups Coconut Yogurt

4 Cloves Garlic, minced

1 Teaspoon Fresh Ginger, grated

Sea Salt

1 Package Extra-Firm Tofu, cubed

1/2 Cup Vegan Butter

1 Teaspoon Cumin Seeds

1 Onion, diced

2 Teaspoons Garam Masala

2 Teaspoons Curry Powder

1 Teaspoon Paprika

1 Teaspoon Cinnamon

2 Teaspoons Cayenne (optional

1 6 Ounce Can Tomato Paste

1 14 Ounce Can Coconut Milk

1 Cup Vegetable Broth

Cilantro, for garnish

Cooked Jasmine or Basmati Rice

Naan (optional

Directions:

In a bowl, make a marinade by mixing coconut yogurt, garlic, ginger, and sea salt. Add tofu and toss to coat. Refrigerate for 1 hour.

After marinade is ready, spread out tofu in a single layer on a baking sheet. Broil until tofu starts to turn brown on all sides, about 20 minutes, turning tofu ever 5 minutes. Set aside when done.

Turn on the instant pot to saute mode and melt butter.

Add cumin seeds and cook for 1 minute.

Add onions and cook until soft (2-3 minutes

Add garam masala, curry powder, paprika, cinnamon, and cayenne (optional). Stir.

Stir in tomato paste, coconut milk, and broth.

Set instant pot to manual mode and cook for 12 minutes.

When finished, let pressure naturally release for 5 minutes, then quick release.

Stir in tofu.

Top tofu and sauce over rice and garnish with cilantro and serve with naan (optional

Enjoy!

192.   Thai Coconut Rice

Preparation Time: 30 MINS| Servings: 4

Ingredients:

1 Cup White Sticky Rice or Jasmine Rice, rinsed

1 1/2 Cups Water

1 14 Ounce Can Coconut Milk

1/2 Teaspoon Sea Salt

1/2 Teaspoon Organic Cane Sugar

Sesame Seeds (optional

Directions:

Add 2 cups of water to inner pot and insert trivet.

In an oven-safe bowl add rice and 1 1/2 cups of water.

Place bowl on trivet, close lid and seal. Pressure cook on high for 15 minutes.

On a stovetop, simmer coconut milk, sugar, and salt.

When rice is done cooking, allow pressure to release naturally then quick release.

Open and remove bowl.

Pour half of the coconut sauce into the rice and stir well.

Top with sesame seeds(optionaland more coconut sauce.

Enjoy!

193. Cauliflower Alfredo

Preparation Time: 25 MINS| Servings: 6

Ingredients:

2 Tablespoons Vegan Butter

1/2 Onion, chopped

4 Cloves Garlic, minced

1 Cup Vegetable

1 head cauliflower, stem and leaves removed, chopped

2 Teaspoons Garlic Powder

Sea Salt

1/4 Cup Plain Unsweetened Almond Milk

1 Package Pasta (fettuccini, linguini, or spaghetti

Sun-Dried Tomatoes (optional

Fresh Parsley (Optional

Directions:

On saute mode on instant pot, melt vegan butter. Saute onion and minced garlic for 2-3 minutes.

Add broth and cauliflower.

Cover the pot and seal it.

Set to manual for 6 minutes.

On a stovetop, cook pasta according to package directions. Set aside.

When instant pot is done cooking, allow to naturally release pressure for 10 minutes, then quick release.

Use an immersion blender to blend ingredients or puree with a standard blender.

Add garlic powder and sea salt. Blend. Taste and add more garlic and salt to taste.

One tablespoon at a time, add almond milk to desired consistency.

Serve with pasta and top with sun-dried tomatoes and fresh parsley (optional

Enjoy!

194.   Spaghetti Squash

Preparation Time: 12 MINS| Servings: 3

Ingredients:

1 Cup Water

1 Spaghetti Squash, washed, halved, and seeds removed

Directions:

Place the metal tripod (trivetinto the instant pot and 1 cup of water.

Put one squash on top of the other with cut sides facing up.

Close the lid and seal.

Cook in manual mode, high pressure, for 5 minutes.

Let the pressure release for 5 minutes. Quick release and open.

Shred the squash with a fork to see if it is done. If it does not shred easily, cook on high pressure for an additional 1-2 minutes.

Serve with favorite store bought pasta sauce or drizzle with olive oil and fresh garlic

Enjoy!

195. Butternut Squash Risotto

Preparation Time: 20 MINS| Servings: 8

Ingredients:

3 Tablespoons Extra Virgin Olive Oil

1 1/2 Pound Butternut Squash, peeled, halved, seeds removed and cubed

2 Teaspoons Ground Sage

Sea Salt and Black Pepper

1 Onion, diced

5 1/2 Cups Vegetable Broth

4 Tablespoons Vegan Butter

2 1/2 Cups Arborio Rice

1 Cup Dry White Wine (optional

1 Tablespoon Nutritional Yeast (optional

Directions:

On saute feature, heat olive oil and add squash, sage, salt, and pepper. Cook for 9 minutes.

Add onion and cook for 1 minute.

Add vegan butter, wine(optionaland broth. Stir to combine.

Add rice and stir.

Close the lid and seal.

On manual mode, set time to 5 minutes.

When done, quick release.

Stir in the nutritional yeast and allow to sit for 5 minutes to thicken.

Serve warm. Enjoy!

196. Sweet Potatoes

Preparation Time: 29 MINS| Servings: 4

Ingredients:

4 Sweet Potatoes, scrubbed and rinsed

1 1/2 Cups Water

Optional Toppings:

Scrambled Tofu, Avocado, Tomatoes

Vegan Butter, Coconut Sugar, Cinnamon

Arugula, Olive Oil, Lemon, Sea Salt

Directions:

Add water to the instant pot.

Place the steaming tray inside and put potatoes on top.

Cover with lid and seal.

Pressure cook for 18 minutes on manual mode.

When done cooking, allow pressure to release on its own (about 15 minutes).

Remove lid.

Serve immediately with desired toppings. Enjoy!

197. Asian Dumplings

Preparation Time: 32 MINS| Servings: 12 Dumplings

Ingredients:

1 1/12 Tablespoons Sesame Oil

3 Cloves Garlic, minced

1 Tablespoon Fresh Ginger, minced

1 Cup Mushrooms, minced

1/2 Cup Tamari Sauce, Soy Sauce, or Coconut Aminos(for soy free

1 Teaspoon Sriracha

1 Tablespoon Rice Vinegar

1 Tablespoon Sesame Seeds

12 Vegan Dumpling Wrappers

1 1/2 Cups Water(for steaming

Directions

On saute mode, heat the sesame oil. When hot, add garlic and ginger. Cook for 1 minute.

Add mushrooms and saute until juices are released from mushrooms.

Add tamari, soy sauce, or coconut aminos, sriracha, rice vinegar, and sesame seeds. Saute until all liquid is cooked out.

Prepare a small bowl of water. Lay out a wrapper and spread water around the edge with fingers.

Fill each dumpling with 1 tablespoon of filling in the middle of the wrapper and press edges together to seal. Place each dumpling onto the vegetable steamer that is lightly coated with oil.

After all wrappers are made, remove the liner from instant pot and add water.

Place the vegetable steamer filled with dumplings into instant pot. Cover with lid and seal. Select the steam option and set to 7 minutes.

When done, open steam release valve manually.

Serve immediately with tamari sauce, soy sauce, coconut aminos, or sriracha for dipping.

Enjoy!

198. Jackfruit Tamales

Preparation Time: 1 Hour, 45 MINS| Servings: 10

Ingredients:

10-15 Corn Husks

1 Tablespoon Olive Oil

1 Onion, chopped

1 Tablespoon Garlic, minced

2 Teaspoons Cumin

1/2 Teaspoon Chili Powder

4 Cups Vegetable Broth, plus 1/2 Cup for jackfruit filling

1 20 Ounce Can Green Jackfruit, drained

4 Cups Masa Harina Flour

2 Teaspoons Baking Powder

1 Teaspoon Sea Salt, plus more to taste for jackfruit filling

1 Cup Coconut Oil, melted

Directions:

Soak the corn husks in hot water in the sink for 1 hour.

On the stovetop, heat 1 tablespoon olive oil, add onions, garlic, cumin, and chili powder. Cook until onions are soft.

Add 1/2 cup of broth. Stir until combined.

Add jackfruit and simmer for a few minutes stirring occasionally.

Shred jackfruit and cook for 5 minutes or until liquid had cooked down.

In a bowl, whisk masa harina, baking powder, and sea salt. Then add coconut oil.

Add the broth 1/4 cup at a time until dough is soft and spongy, but not sticky.

One at a time, remove corn husk from sink and lay on a flat surface and spread out a scoop of masa into the middle of the husk about 1/4 inch thick.

Place a spoonful of jackfruit mixture onto the masa and take the two sides of the husk and let the masa surround the filling, then roll. Fold over one end and secure with a strip of the corn husk.

Pour 2 cups of water into the instant pot and insert the steam rack.

Vertically line the tamales around the instant pot with the open side up.

When the pot is filled, place a corn husk on top.

Close the lid and seal.

Cook on manual setting 40 minutes on low pressure.

They are done with the tamale easily separates from the corn husk. Cook for 10 more minutes if needed.

Remove steamer and allow to cool a little uncovered for up to 10 minutes.

Enjoy!

199.   Red Beans and Rice

Preparation Time: 55 MINS| Servings: 6

Ingredients:

1 Pound Seitan (optional

1/4 Cup Olive oil

1 Large Onion, diced

1 Celery Rib, chopped

1 Large Bell Pepper, diced

2 Tablespoons Garlic, minced

Sea Salt and Pepper

2 Teaspoons Paprika

2 Teaspoons Store Bought Cajun Seasoning

1 Sprig Fresh Thyme

2 Bay Leaves

1 Pound Dry Red Kidney Beans, thoroughly rinsed

7 Cups Vegetable Broth or Water

3 Cups Cooked Brown Rice

Directions:

On saute setting, add olive oil. When hot, add onion, celery, bell pepper, and garlic. Cook for 2-3 minutes or until soft.

Add salt and pepper, paprika, cajun seasoning, thyme, and bay leaves. Stir well for 1 minute.

Add beans and broth or water. Stir.

Cover, seal, and set to manual on high pressure for 28 minutes.

During this time, cook rice on stove top.

When time is up, quick release and remove lid.

If using seitan, add at this time, cover and seal again. Cook for another 15 minutes on manual setting at high pressure. Allow pressure to release on its own when done cooking.

Serve hot over rice. Enjoy!

200.   Teriyaki Seitan Cauliflower Rice Bowl

Preparation Time: 15 MINS| Servings: 4

Ingredients:

1 Tablespoon Sesame Oil

1 Clove Garlic, minced

1/2 Inch Ginger Root, peeled, minced

1 Pound Seitan or 1 Package Extra Firm Tofu

1/2 Cup Vegetable Broth

4 Cups Cauliflower Florets

1/4 Cup Store Bought Teriyaki Sauce

2 Cups Edamame, shelled and cooked (frozen and thawed is okay

1 Avocado, sliced

4 Green Onions, chopped

Sesame Seeds(optional

Extra Teriyaki Sauce(optional

Directions:

On Saute setting, add sesame oil. When oil is hot, cook garlic and ginger until brown about 30 seconds to 1 minute.

Add the seitan or tofu and cook for 1-2 minutes then add broth.

Place the steaming basket over the seitan and add the cauliflower florets to the basket. Close the lid and seal.

Cook on high pressure for 1 minute, then quick release when done.

Remove the steaming basket. Also, remove the remaining contents of seitan or tofu and liquid from the instant pot to a separate container or bowl.

Add the cauliflower back to the bottom of the instant pot and use a mash potato masher to break down the cauliflower into rice.

To the seitan or tofu, add teriyaki sauce and stir until combined well.

Top cauliflower with seitan or tofu, edamame, avocado, green onions, sesame seeds(optional), and extra teriyaki sauce(optional). Serve immediately and enjoy!

201. Pasta With Mushroom Tomato Sauce

Preparation Time: 15 MINS| Servings: 5

Ingredients:

5-6 Cups Mushrooms, chopped

1/4 Cup Onion, diced

2 Cloves Garlic, minced

1 Teaspoon Dried Basil

1 Teaspoon Dried Parsley

1 Teaspoon Dried Oregano

3/4 Teaspoon Sea Salt

1 Jar 25.5 Ounces Pasta Sauce

2 Cups Water

1 Package or 8 Ounces Whole Wheat or Gluten-Free Pasta

Directions:

On saute mode add mushrooms, onions, garlic, dried basil, parsley, oregano, and sea salt. Mushrooms will release liquid as they cook down. Cook 3-4 minutes.

Add sauce, water, and pasta. All ingredients should be covered in liquid. Add more water if needed to cover all ingredients.

Place lid on instant pot and cook on manual mode on high pressure for 9 minutes.

Quick release when time is done.

Serve hot. Enjoy!

202.   Fragrant Vegetable Rice

Preparation Time: 29 MINS| Servings: 4

Ingredients:

3 Tablespoons Sesame Oil

2 Teaspoons Fresh Ginger, grated or minced

1 Tablespoon Sesame Seeds

1 Clove Garlic, minced

1 Yellow Onion, chopped

1/2 Pound Fresh Asparagus, trimmed and cut into 1-inch pieces

1 Bell Pepper, chopped

2 Cups Mushrooms, sliced

3 Tablespoons Tamari or Soy Sauce

1 Tablespoon Vegan Butter

1 1/2 Cups Water

3/4 Cups Jasmine or Basmati Rice

Directions:

Add two tablespoons of sesame oil to instant pot. On the saute setting, cook ginger, sesame seeds, and garlic for 1 minute.

Add onions and cook for 1 minute.

Add bell pepper, asparagus, and mushrooms. Cook for 2 minutes.

Add tamari or soy sauce and vegan butter. Stir to combine.

Mix in rice and water and stir well.

Cover the instant pot and seal. Pressure cook for 4 minutes.

When done allow to naturally release for 10 minutes.

Serve hot. Enjoy!

203.   Mexican Quinoa Bowl

Preparation Time: 25 MINS| Servings: 2

Ingredients:

1 Cup Quinoa

1 Cup Salsa, any store brand

1 Cup Water

1 15 Ounce Can Black Beans, thoroughly drained and rinsed

2 Cups Corn Kernels, thawed if using frozen

Sea Salt and Pepper

1 Lime, zested and juiced

1/2 Cup Cilantro, chopped

1 Romaine Lettuce Heart, chopped

1/2 Pint Grape Tomatoes, sliced lengthwise

1/2 Cup Red Onion, diced

1 Avocado, sliced

Directions:

Add quinoa, salsa, water, beans, corn, sea salt, and pepper to instant pot. Close lid and seal.

Press the Rice button or cook on manual setting for 12 minutes on low pressure. When done cooking, allow pressure to release on its own.

Remove lid and fluff quinoa with a fork.

Add lime zest and juice, cilantro, and more salt and pepper if needed. Toss well.

Serve warm and top with lettuce, tomatoes, red onion, and avocado.

Enjoy!

204.   Mac And Cheese

Preparation Time: 13 MINS| Servings: 4-6

Ingredients:

1 Pound Dry Macaroni or any dry short pasta

4 Cups Water

1 1/2 Cups Unsweetened Plain Almond Milk

2 Tablespoons All Purpose Flour or Tapioca Starch

2-3 Cups Shredded Vegan Cheese

Sea Salt

2 Tablespoons Vegan Butter

2 Tablespoons Mustard Powder or Nutritional Yeast

Directions:

Add macaroni or other dry pasta, water, and salt to instant pot.

Close lid and seal.

On the manual setting, set to 4 minutes.

While instant pot is cooking, whisk almond milk and flour or tapioca starch until combined. Set aside.

When done, quick release valve and open when steam is gone.

Turn instant pot on saute mode.

Stir in almond milk and flour mixture, vegan butter, cheese, mustard powder or nutritional yeast. Stir well.

When the cheese is melted, turn off instant pot, taste and add more salt if needed, serve and enjoy!

205. Refried Beans

Preparation Time: 55 MINS| Servings: 8

Ingredients:

1 Tablespoon Olive Oil

1 Cup Onions, diced

3 Cloves Garlic, minced

1 Jalapeno, seeds removed and minced

Sea Salt

Pinch Cayenne Pepper(optional

1 pound dry Black or Pinto Beans, thoroughly rinsed

6 Cups Vegetable Broth or Water

1 Teaspoon Cumin

1 Tablespoon Chili Powder

1 Teaspoon Oregano

Fresh Cilantro, Chopped

Directions:

On the saute setting, heat oil and add onions, garlic, jalapenos, and sea salt and cayenne pepper(optional). Cook for 3-4 minutes until soft and browned.

Add beans, vegetable broth or water, cumin, chili powder, and oregano to the instant pot. Cover with lid and secure.

On the bean/chili mode, cook for 45 minutes or manual mode, high pressure for 35 minutes.

When done, allow the pressure to release naturally or use quick release.

Reserve 2 1/2 cups of liquid and drain the rest.

Use a potato masher and mash to desired consistency. If using a blender, add beans and blend with reserved liquid.

Stir in cilantro. Serve warm. Enjoy!

206.   Mushroom Marsala Rotini

Preparation Time: 25 MINS| Servings: 4

Ingredients:

3 Tablespoons Olive Oil

1 Small Onion, diced

4 Cloves Garlic, chopped

1/2 Pound Fresh Mushrooms, sliced

Sea Salt and Pepper

2 Tablespoons All-Purpose Flour

1/2 Cup Marsala Wine

1 1/4 Teaspoon Better Than Bouillon No Beef Base Vegetarian

1 1/2 Cups Water

2 Tablespoons Vegan Butter

Directions:

On saute mode, add olive oil, when hot add onions, garlic, mushrooms, and season with sea salt. Cook for 3-4 minutes stirring frequently until fragrant.

Stir in flour and cook 1 minute.

Add wine to deglaze pot.

Add No Beef Base, water, and vegan butter. Stir to combine.

Turn pot on to manual mode, seal, and set to 5 minutes.

Quick release and uncover.

Turn on saute mode and stir until sauce becomes desired consistency.

Enjoy!

207. Seitan with Apple Brandy Gravy

Preparation Time: 50 Minutes

Servings: 4

Ingredients:

4 chicken-flavored seitan breasts

2 apples, peeled and sliced

1/4 cup brandy

1 3/4 cups apple cider

2 tablespoons olive oil

1 small onion, chopped

1 1/2 tablespoons vegan chicken-flavored bouillon

2 cloves garlic, minced

1 teaspoon dried thyme

1/8 teaspoon cinnamon

1/8 teaspoon nutmeg

Salt and pepper, to taste

3 tablespoons flour

Directions:

Heat the olive oil on the sauté setting and cook the onion for 5 minutes. Add the garlic and cook an additional minute.

Add the rest of the ingredients, except for the flour. Seal the lid and cook on high 4 minutes. Let the pressure release naturally, then remove the lid and switch to sauté setting.

Remove the seitan and cover it with foil to keep warm. Whisk in 2 to 3 tablespoons of flour to thicken the sauce and simmer for 30 minutes.

Add the seitan to reheat in the sauce for a few minutes right before you are ready to serve. Serve with a baked potato.

208. Kalamata Olive Seitan

Preparation Time: 15 Minutes

Servings: 4

Ingredients:

6 chicken-flavored seitan breasts

1 cup pitted and sliced Kalamata olives

1 stalk celery, minced

10 ounces grape tomatoes, halved

1 cup red wine

1 tablespoon tomato paste

1/2 cup water

1/2 teaspoon fennel seeds, crushed

1/4 teaspoon ground thyme

2 cloves garlic, minced

1/2 teaspoon fresh ground pepper

Directions:

Spray the instant pot with nonstick spray. Combine all the ingredients.

Seal the lid and cook on high 4 minutes, then allow pressure to release naturally. Serve with a leafy green salad.

209. Italian Mushroom Tofu Strata

Preparation Time: 12 Minutes

Servings: 4

Ingredients:

8ounces Italian bread, toasted, diced

½cup chopped roasted red bell pepper

2cups crumbled firm tofu

2tablespoons nutritional yeast

8ounces cremini mushrooms, chopped

½teaspoon onion powder

¼teaspoon ground turmeric

Salt and black pepper

½teaspoon dried basil

3plum tomatoes, chopped

2teaspoons olive oil (optional

1cup vegetable broth1onion, minced

3garlic cloves, minced

½cup chopped fresh basil

2medium-size zucchini, thinly sliced

Directions:

Add the yeast, tofu, onion, basil, seasoning, turmeric and broth in a blender.

Blend until smooth.

Combine the bell pepper, tomatoes and basil in a bowl.

In another bowl combine the zucchini, garlic, mushroom and bread.

Add half the tomato mixture into your instant pot.

Then add the zucchini mixture. Add the remaining tomato mixture on top of the zucchini mixture.

Finally add the tofu mixture on top

Cook with the lid on for about 8 minutes.

Serve hot.

210. Cajun Vegan Shrimps

Preparation Time: 10 Minutes

Servings: 6

Ingredients:

½ cup coconut oil

½ cup chopped onion

½ cup chopped carrots

10oz. vegan shrimps

1 green bell pepper, seeded, chopped

¼ cup all-purpose flour

1 cup water

4 tablespoons lemon juice

Salt and pepper, to taste

3 cloves garlic

2 teaspoons Cajun seasoning

¼ cup chopped cilantro

4 cups cooked brown rice, to serve with

Directions:

Heat coconut oil in Instant pot on Sauté.

Add vegetables and cook 5 minutes.

Sprinkle veggies with flour and cook 1 minute.

Add water and stir until smooth.

Add remaining ingredients, except the rice, and season to taste.

Cover and select Manual.

High-pressure 4 minutes.

Use a quick pressure release method.

Serve over rice.

211. Seitan Delicacy

Preparation Time: 15 Minutes

Servings: 6

Ingredients:

2 tablespoons vegetable oil

1 tablespoon tomato puree

2 cups vegetable stock

2 cups red wine

1lb. cooked and sliced seitan

1 cup carrots, sliced

½ cup onion, sliced

2 tablespoons all-purpose flour

Salt and pepper, to taste

2 cups sliced brown mushrooms

1 bay leaf

2 cloves garlic, minced

1 ½ cup peeled pearl onions

1 tablespoon coconut oil

1 teaspoon dried thyme

Directions:

Heat oil into Instant Pot on Sauté.

Add onions and carrots. Cook 5 minutes.

Add garlic and spices. Cook 1 minute. Sprinkle with flour and cook 1 minute.

Pour in stock and simmer 2 minutes.

Toss in remaining ingredients.

Lock lid into place and select Manual.

High-pressure 8 minutes.

Use a natural pressure release method.

Serve warm.

212. Stuffed Peppers

 Preparation Time: 25 Minutes

Servings: 5

Ingredients:

5 bell peppers, seeds removed

1 medium-sized onion, peeled and finely chopped

7 oz button mushrooms, sliced

4 garlic cloves, peeled and crushed

4 tbsp of extra-virgin olive oil

1 tsp of salt

¼ tsp of freshly ground black pepper

¼ cup of rice

½ tbsp. of cayenne pepper

Directions:

Use package instructions to pre-cook the rice, or simply place ¼ cup of rice in 1 cup of water and bring it to a boil. Cook for 10 minutes.

With the cooker's lid off, heat up two tablespoons of olive oil and place the onion and crushed garlic in the stainless steel insert. Press "Sautee" and stir-fry until translucent and add mushrooms, salt, pepper, and cayenne pepper.

Mix well and continue to cook until the water evaporates. Remove from the heat and combine with rice.

Using a wooden spoon, combine the ingredients and add the remaining olive oil.

Use the mixture to stuff the pepper and gently transfer them to your instant pot.

Securely lock the lid and press "Manual" button. Set the timer for 10 minutes and adjust the steam release handle. Cook on high pressure.

When done, press "Cancel" button and release the steam naturally.

Enjoy!

213. Eggplant Caponata

 Preparation Time: 42 Minutes

Servings: 8

Ingredients:

4-5 eggplants, sliced

2 medium-sized onions, peeled and chopped

10 large, fresh tomatoes, roughly chopped

7.5 oz green olives

7.5 oz capers

1 medium-sized chili pepper

2 stalks of celery

½ cup of oil

3 tablespoons of red wine vinegar

Salt to taste

1 tsp of sugar

½ tbsp of basil, dry

Directions:

Chop the eggplants into bite-sized pieces and season with some salt. Allow it to stand for about 30 minutes and rinse well.

Plug in your instant pot and add the eggplants in the stainless steel insert. Add all the remaining ingredients and securely close the lid. Adjust the steam release handle and press "Manual" button. Set the timer for 12 minutes and cook on high pressure.

When done, press "Cancel" button and release the pressure naturally.

Open the pot and serve warm.

214. Potato Mushrooms Pot

Preparation Time: 15 Minutes

Servings: 6

Ingredients:

2 tablespoons vegetable oil

½ lb. potatoes, peeled, cubed

1lb. sliced shiitake mushrooms

1lb. sliced cremini mushrooms

4 cups vegetable stock

4 cloves garlic, minced

Salt and pepper, to taste

1 lb. sliced oyster mushrooms

½ cup red wine

1 tablespoon coconut aminos

¼ cup chopped onion

1 teaspoon thyme

Directions:

Heat vegetable oil into Instant pot on Sauté.

Add onions and cook 4 minutes.

Add garlic and cook 1 minute.

Stir in mushrooms and cook 1 minute.

Add remaining ingredients.

Lock lid into place and select Manual.

High-pressure 9 minutes.

Use a quick pressure release method.

Serve warm.

215.   Black Bean, Chorizo & Enchilada Lasagna

Preparation Time: 15 Minutes

Servings: 6

Ingredients:

12 ounces soy chorizo

1 medium-size sweet potato, thinly sliced

1 can black beans

2 cups enchilada sauce

1 package corn tortillas

1/4 teaspoon cumin

1/4 teaspoon chili powder

Directions:

Season the chorizo with cumin and chili powder.

Oil the instant pot and pour a quarter of the sauce into the bottom. Add a single layer of tortilla, then add a third of the chorizo, sweet potatoes, and black beans. Repeat the layers, finishing with one more layer of tortillas and sauce.

Seal the lid and cook on high 4 minutes. Serve with vegan sour cream for garnish.

216. Yellow Split Pea with Lemon

Preparation Time: 40 Minutes

Servings: 5

Ingredients:

2 cups split yellow peas

1 cup onions, finely chopped

1 large carrot, sliced

2 large potatoes, chopped

3 tbsp olive oil

¼ cup freshly squeezed lemon juice

3 garlic cloves, crushed

1 tsp cayenne pepper

½ tsp salt

4 cups vegetable stock

Directions:

Plug in your instant pot and press the "Sautee" button. Heat up the olive oil in the stainless steel insert and add onions. Stir-fry for one minute. Add the remaining vegetables and continue to cook for 5-6 minutes. Stir in the cayenne pepper and season with salt.

Finally, pour in the vegetable stock and close the lid. Set the steam release handle and set the "Manual" mode for 25 minutes.

When done, press "Cancel" button and perform a quick release. Open the lid and stir in the lemon juice.

Serve immediately.

217. Spicy White Peas

 Preparation Time: 30 Minutes

Servings: 4

Ingredients:

1 lb of white peas

4 slices of vegan bacon

1 large onion, finely chopped

1 small chili pepper, finely chopped

2 tbsp of all-purpose flour

2 tbsp of coconut oil

1 tbsp of cayenne pepper

3 bay leaves, dried

1 tsp of salt

½ tsp of freshly ground black pepper

Directions:

Plug in your instant pot and press "Sautee" button. Melt the coconut oil in the stainless steel insert. Add chopped onion and stir-fry until translucent.

Add bacon, peas, finely chopped chili pepper, bay leaves, salt, and pepper. Gently stir in two tablespoons of flour and add 3 cups of water.

Close the lid and set the steam release handle. Press "Manual" button and set the timer for 15 minutes. Cook on high pressure.

When done, press "Cancel" button and release the steam naturally. Turn off the instant pot.

Let it chill for 10 minutes before serving.

Enjoy!

218. Stuffed Potatoes

 Preparation Time: 60 Minutes

Servings: 3

Ingredients:

6 small potatoes, whole

¼ cup olive oil

3 garlic cloves, crushed

¼ cup crumbled tofu

1 tsp fresh rosemary, finely chopped

½ tsp dried thyme

2 oz button mushrooms, sliced

1 tsp salt

Directions:

Rinse well the potatoes and drain in a large colander. Rub with salt and place in your instant pot.

Add enough water to cover and seal the lid. Press "Manual" button and set the timer for 30 minutes.

When you hear the cooker's end signal, perform a quick release and open. Gently remove the potatoes and chill for a while keeping them whole.

Meanwhile, in a medium-sized bowl, combine olive oil with crushed garlic, tofu, rosemary, thyme, and mushrooms. Press the "Sautee" button and add the mixture. Gently simmer until mushrooms soften and cheese melts. Remove from the cooker.

Now, cut the top of each potato and spoon out the middle. Fill with tofu mixture and serve immediately.

Enjoy!

219. Seitan with Tomatillo Sauce

Preparation Time: 15 Minutes

Servings: 10

Ingredients:

4 cups cubed chicken-flavored seitan

1 2/3 pounds tomatillos, husked and chopped

1 can green chilis

3 cloves garlic, minced

1/4 cup apple cider vinegar

1 teaspoon salt

2 teaspoons chili powder

1/2 teaspoon cumin

1/4 teaspoon coriander

1 teaspoon olive oil

1/4 cup water

Juice of 1 lime

Directions:

Add everything except the seitan to a food processor and blend to make the sauce.

Add the sauce and the seitan to the instant pot. Seal the lid and cook on high 4 minutes, then let the pressure release naturally.

Serve in warm tortillas or over a bed of rice.

220. Garlic Shiitake

 Preparation Time: 45 Minutes

Servings: 4

Ingredients:

1 lb shiitake mushrooms

2 large potatoes, finely chopped

4 garlic cloves, crushed

2 tbsp oil

1 tsp garlic powder

1 tbsp cumin seeds

½ tsp chili powder

1 large zucchini, chopped

1 cup onions

2 cups vegetable stock

1 cup tomato sauce

Directions:

With the cooker's lid off, heat up the olive oil on the "Sautee" mode. Add cumin seeds and stir-fry for one minute. Now, add onions, chili powder, crushed garlic, and garlic powder. Cook for 3 minutes, stirring constantly.

Add mushrooms and continue to cook on "Sautee" mode for 3 minutes.

Finally, add the remaining ingredients and seal the lid. Press the "Manual" button and set the timer for 20 minutes.

When done, press "Cancel" button and release the steam pressure naturally.

Open the lid and serve immediately.

Enjoy!

221. Stuffed Bell Peppers

Preparation Time: 35 Minutes

Servings: 4

Ingredients:

5 bell peppers, seeds removed

1 medium-sized onion, peeled and finely chopped

7oz button mushrooms, sliced

4 garlic cloves, peeled and crushed

4 tbsp of extra-virgin olive oil

1 tsp of salt

¼ tsp of freshly ground black pepper

¼ cup of rice

½ tbsp. of Cayenne pepper

2 cups vegetable stock

Directions:

With the cooker's lid off, heat up two tablespoons of olive oil on the "Sautee" mode. Add onions and garlic and stir-fry until translucent. Press the "Cancel" button and set aside.

Rinse well each bell pepper and pat dry with some kitchen paper. Remove the stem along with seeds.

In a small bowl, combine rice with the mixture from your pot. Add mushrooms and stir all well. Season with salt, pepper, and cayenne pepper. Stuff each bell pepper with this mixture. Gently place them in your instant pot, filled side up, and pour in the broth.

Seal the lid and set the steam release handle. Press the "Manual" mode and set the timer for 15 minutes.

When done, press "Cancel" button and release the pressure naturally.

Enjoy!

222. Ginger Stew

Preparation Time: 35 Minutes

Servings: 4

Ingredients:

2 cups green peas

1 large onion, chopped

4 cloves of garlic, finely chopped

3 ½ oz of olives, pitted

1 tbsp of ginger, ground

1 tbsp of turmeric, ground

1 tbsp of salt

4 cups of vegetable stock

3 tbsp olive oil

Directions:

Rinse well the green peas using a large colander. Drain and set aside.

Plug in your instant pot and press "Sautee" button. Heat up the olive oil in the stainless steel insert and add onions and garlic. Stir-fry for 2-3 minutes, or until translucent.

Now, add the remaining ingredients and close the lid. Set the steam release handle and press "Stew" button.

When you hear the cooker's end signal, perform a quick release.

Open the pot and serve immediately.

223. Chickpeas with Onions

 Preparation Time: 35 Minutes

Servings: 5

Ingredients:

1 lb chickpeas, soaked

3 large purple onions, peeled and sliced

2 large tomatoes, roughly chopped

3 oz parsley, chopped

2 cups vegetable broth

1 tbsp cayenne pepper

3 tbsp almond butter

2 tbsp olive oil

1 tsp salt

½ tsp freshly ground black pepper

Directions:

Plug in your instant pot and heat up the oil in the stainless steel insert. Press the "Sautee" button and add onions. Stir-fry for five minutes. Now, add soaked chickpeas, chopped tomatoes, chopped parsley, and vegetable broth. Stir in the cayenne pepper, salt, and freshly ground black pepper.

Close the lid and set the steam release handle. Press the "Stew" button and cook for 30 minutes.

When done, press "Cancel" button and turn off the pot. Perform a quick release and open the pot.

Serve chickpeas warm.

224. Portobello Mushrooms with Green Peas

Preparation Time: 65 Minutes

Servings: 4

Ingredients:

8 oz Portobello mushrooms, sliced

1 cup green peas

1 cup pearl onions, minced

2 large carrots

½ cup celery stalks, chopped

2 garlic cloves, crushed

2 large potatoes, chopped

1 tbsp apple cider vinegar

1 tsp rosemary

1 tbsp cayenne pepper

1 tsp salt

½ tsp pepper, freshly ground

2 tbsp almond butter

3 cups vegetable stock

Directions:

Set your instant pot to "Sautee" mode. Add onions, carrots, celery stalks, and garlic. Sprinkle with some salt, pepper, rosemary, and cayenne pepper. Stir-fry for a few minutes.

Now, add the remaining ingredients and seal the lid. Set the steam release handle and press the "Manual" mode. Set the timer for 30 minutes.

When done, press "Cancel" button and release the pressure naturally.

Open the lid and serve immediately.

225. Lentil Stew

Preparation Time: 35 Minutes

Servings: 4

Ingredients:

1 cup red lentils, soaked

1 medium-sized onion, peeled and finely chopped

½ cup sweet carrot puree

1 tbsp all-purpose flour

½ tsp freshly ground black pepper

½ tsp cumin, ground

½ tsp salt

2 tbsp olive oil

Directions:

Soak the lentils overnight.

Rinse well the lentils under cold running water using a large colander. Drain well and set aside.

Plug in your instant pot and grease the stainless steel insert with olive oil. Press "Sautee" button and heat it up. Add onions and flour. Cook for 10 minutes, stirring constantly.

Now, add the remaining ingredients and pour in about 4 cups of water. Close the lid and set the release steam handle. Press "Manual" button and cook for 30 minutes on high pressure.

Press "Cancel" button and release the steam handle. Turn off the pot and set aside to chill for a while before serving.

Optionally, sprinkle with cayenne pepper and parsley.

226. One Pot Quinoa

 Preparation Time: 20 Minutes

Servings: 2

Ingredients:

4 cups water

2 cups quinoa

3 garlic cloves, minced

2 tbsp rice vinegar

2 tbsp soy sauce

1tsp grated ginger

2 tbsp sugar

8 oz bag of frozen vegetables (Asian-style

Directions:

Combine all the ingredients (except for frozen vegetablesin Instant Pot. Cover the pot with lid. Set steam release handle to 'sealing' and set Instant Pot to manual to 1 minute over high pressure.

Once done, allow it to naturally release pressure for 10 minutes. Change steam release handle to 'venting' to release any remaining steam. Open the lid. Then add thawed frozen veggies and mix well.

227. Instant Pot Hot Dogs

 Preparation Time: 35 Minutes

Servings: 4

Ingredients:

For Marinade:

¼ cup soy sauce

¼ cup water

1 tbsp rice vinegar

½ tsp liquid smoke

½ tsp garlic powder

½ tsp onion powder

For Topping:

Ketchup, mustard, etc

For Hot Dog:

4 large carrots

4 oil-free vegan hot dog buns

Directions:

Place trivet in the inner pot. Pour in 1½ cups water. Place 4 carrots on a trivet and cover the pot with lid. Switch the manual button for 3 minutes over high pressure. Set steam release handle to 'sealing'.

When the timer beeps, change the steam release handle to 'venting' to release the steam immediately.

Mix the marinade ingredients together in a container. Add carrots along with the marinade. Let it marinade for 24 hours.

Take them from marinade and transfer them to Instant Pot. Pour in marinade and switch on sauté button. Switch adjust button to get 'high' temperature setting. Sauté it for 10 minutes.

Serve carrot dogs over desired oil-free hot dog buns topped with favorite sauces.

228. Curried Potato and Cauliflower (Indian Aloo Gobi

Preparation Time: 40 Minutes

Servings: 2

Ingredients:

1 head cauliflower

1½ lbs potatoes, peeled and then chopped

2 cups water

1 red onion, chopped finely

1 tsp salt

3 garlic cloves, minced

 1 tsp ground coriander

1 tsp garam masala

1 tsp chili powder

1/2 tsp turmeric

1 tsp grated ginger

Directions:

Steam the cauliflower head in Instant Pot for 2 minutes on a trivet with 1½ cups water. Immediately release pressure and take out trivet out from Instant Pot. Allow it to cool. Empty the pot of water.

Sauté onions, ginger and garlic for 5 minutes along with ½ cup water (using the sauté function). Once timer beeps, switch on 'Keep Warm/Cancel' button. Add 1½ cups water to the inner pot. Add potatoes and all spices. Mix everything around using a spoon.

Cover the pot with lid and switch on manual button for 8 minutes over high pressure. Set steam release handle to 'sealing'. Once finished cooking, allow pressure to release naturally for about 5-10 minutes. In the meanwhile, chop cauliflower into bite-size bits.

Using the steam release handle to release remaining steam after 5-10 minutes. Add cauliflower pieces and stir around using a spoon.

229. Sloppy Joe in Instant Pot

Preparation Time: 35 Minutes

Servings: 6-8 sloppy joes

Ingredients:

1 cup of red lentils

1 rib of celery, chopped

1 yellow onion, chopped

1/2 of a yellow pepper, chopped

1/2 can (1/2 of an 8 oz canof tomato paste

2 1/2 cups of water

1/4 cup of red wine vinegar

2 tbsp of brown sugar

1 tsp of salt

1 tsp of liquid smoke

3 garlic cloves, minced

2 tbsp of sriracha (optional

1/4 cup of oil-free breadcrumbs

6 or 8 oil-free hamburger buns

Directions:

Except for breadcrumbs and buns, combine all ingredients in Instant Pot. Set steam release handle to 'sealing' and switch on manual button. Cover the pot with lid and set to 15 minutes over high pressure.

Allow the pressure to release naturally for 10-15 minutes. Change steam release handle to 'venting' to release extra steam. Open the lid. Add breadcrumbs and give it a stir.

Serve this sloppy Joe mix over hamburger buns topped with fresh mixed greens, if desired.

230.   Pizza Alla Puttanesca.

 Preparation Time: 15 Minutes

Servings: 6

Ingredients:

Dough:

1½ cups unbleached all-purpose flour

½ cup warm water, or as needed

1 tablespoon olive oil

1½ teaspoons instant yeast

½ teaspoon salt

½ teaspoon Italian seasoning

Sauce:

½ cup crushed tomatoes

½ cup shredded vegan mozzarella cheese

¼ cup pitted green olives, sliced

¼ cup pitted kalamata olives, sliced

1 tablespoon chopped fresh flat-leaf parsley

 1 tablespoon capers, rinsed and drained

¼ teaspoon garlic powder

¼ teaspoon sugar

¼ teaspoon dried basil

¼ teaspoon dried oregano

¼ teaspoon hot red pepper flakes

 Salt and freshly ground black pepper

Directions:

Get a bowl to mix your dough. Whisk together the flour, yeast, salt, and seasoning.

Add the oil slowly whilst stirring, then add water little by little until the dough ball is formed.

Knead the dough on a floured surface for 2 minutes.

Shape it and put it in a warm bowl to rise for an hour.

Whilst the dough rises, mix the sauce. Combine tomatoes, olives, capers, parsley, basil, oregano, garlic powder, sugar, red pepper, salt and pepper.

Oil a tray that will fit in your instant pot and stretch the dough to fit it.

Spread the sauce over the dough.

Insert the tray into your instant pot and cook for 10 minutes on steam.

Release the pressure quickly and sprinkle the mozzarella on top at the end.

231. Seitan Fajitas.

Preparation Time: 40 Minutes

Servings: 6

Ingredients:

1lb seitan, cut into strips

2 tablespoons tomato paste

1½ cups tomato salsa

1 tablespoon chili powder

1 tablespoon soy sauce

2 large bell peppers (any color), seeded and cut into ¼-inch-thick strips

1 large yellow onion, thinly sliced

1 garlic clove, minced

Salt and freshly ground black pepper

2 tablespoons freshly squeezed lime juice

1 ripe Hass avocado, peeled, pitted, and diced, for garnish

1 large ripe tomato, diced, for garnish

Directions:

Mix the tomato paste, salsa, chili powder, and soy sauce until combined well.

Put the bell peppers, onion, and garlic in your instant pot.

Put your seitan strips on top. Try and avoid them touching.

Pour the tomato mix over everything.

Seal and cook on Poultry for 30 minutes.

Depressurize naturally, stir in the lime to taste.

Serve and top with avocado and tomato.

232. Zesty Stuffed Bell Peppers.

 Preparation Time: 30 Minutes

Servings: 4

Ingredients:

4 large bell peppers (any color or a combination

1 (14-ouncecan tomato sauce

2 cups cooked brown or white rice

1½ cups cooked pinto beans or black beans or 1 (15-ouncecan beans, rinsed and drained

1 cup fresh or thawed frozen corn kernels

1 cup diced fresh tomatoes or 1 (14-ouncecan diced tomatoes, drained

2 teaspoons olive oil (optional

4 garlic cloves, minced

4 scallions, chopped

1 tablespoon chili powder

2 teaspoons minced chipotle chiles in adobo

1½ teaspoon ground cumin

1¼ teaspoon dried oregano

½ teaspoon sugar

Salt and freshly ground black pepper

Directions:

Warm the oil in your instant pot, leaving the lid open.

When the oil is hot, add the garlic and scallions and soften for 3 minutes.

Add the chili powder, and a teaspoon of both the cumin and the oregano.

Put the garlic mixture in a bowl to one side. Add the rice, beans, corn, tomatoes, and chiles with a little salt and pepper. Mix well.

Top and hollow your bell peppers.

Fill the peppers evenly with the mix and set them in the steamer basket of your instant pot.

Mix the tomato sauce, remaining cumin, remaining oregano, sugar, and salt in the base of your instant pot.

Lower the steamer basket, seal, and cook on Steam for 24 minutes.

Depressurize fast and serve immediately.

233.   Moroccan Stuffed Peppers

Preparation Time: 30 Minutes

Servings: 4

Ingredients:

4 large bell peppers (assorted colors look great

2 cups boiling water or vegetable broth

2 cups couscous

1 cup cooked chickpeas or 1 (15-ouncecan chickpeas

1 medium-size yellow onion, minced

2 carrots, peeled and minced

1 large zucchini, minced

3 garlic cloves, minced

3 tablespoons tomato paste

2 teaspoons olive oil

2 teaspoons harissa or hot chili paste

2 teaspoons ground coriander

1 teaspoon paprika

1 teaspoon ground cinnamon

½ tablespoon ground cumin

1 teaspoon salt

¼ teaspoon freshly ground black pepper

1 tablespoon minced fresh flat-leaf parsley leaves, for garnish

Directions:

Top and hollow our the peppers. Remove the stems, then chop the tops and keep the diced pepper.

Warm the oil in your instant pot.

When hot, add the onion and soften for 4 minutes.

Add the carrots, pepper tops, zucchini, garlic, and cook for 2 more minutes.

Add the harissa, tomato paste, coriander, cinnamon, cumin, paprika, salt and pepper.

Add the couscous and water, stir well.

Add the chickpeas and stir again.

Pack the stuffing into the peppers and put them in the steamer basket of your instant pot.

Put a cup of water in your instant pot. Lower the steamer basket.

Seal and cook on Steam for 24 minutes.

Depressurize naturally and serve immediately, topped with parsley.

234. Corn Chorizo pie

 Preparation Time: 6 Minutes

Servings: 6

Ingredients:

12 soft corn tortillas

1 crumbled vegan chorizo

1 onion, minced

1 teaspoon olive oil

2canned chipotle chilies in adobo, minced

1½cups corn kernels

1½cups shredded vegan cheddar cheese

2tablespoons chili powder

1tablespoon tomato paste

1tablespoon grated unsweetened dark chocolate

1(15-ouncecan vegan refried beans, stirred

1teaspoon ground cumin

¼teaspoon black pepper

1teaspoon smoked paprika

1teaspoon dark brown sugar

1teaspoon dried oregano

8ounces steamed diced tempeh, chopped seitan

½teaspoon salt

1(14.5-ouncecan crushed tomatoes

4garlic cloves, minced

1½cups cooked pinto beans

Directions:

Add the onion, garlic and oil in the instant pot.

Cook for 30 seconds and then add the tomato paste, cumin, chipotle chiles, chocolate, oregano, chili powder, paprika, brown sugar, and seasoning.

Add some water and cover with lid.

Cook for 2 minutes and then add the tomatoes.

Cover and cook for 1 minute.

Add the tempeh, beans, corn and mix well.

Cover and cook for another 5 minutes.

Serve hot.

235. Cheesy Tomato Gratin

Preparation Time: 10 Minutes

Servings: 6

Ingredients:

1(14.5-ouncecan petite diced tomatoes

1cup shredded vegan mozzarella cheese

3large potatoes, peeled and sliced

½teaspoon smoked paprika

¼cup vegetable broth

1onion, minced

2tablespoons chili powder

½teaspoon ground cumin

¼teaspoon cayenne pepper

3garlic cloves, minced

1teaspoon dried oregano

3tablespoons tomato paste

Salt and black pepper

Directions:

Add the onion, garlic in your instant pot.

Cover and cook for 30 seconds.

Add the broth, oregano, cumin, tomato paste, cayenne, paprika and chili powder.

Add the tomatoes, and mix well.

Cook for 2 minutes.

Add the potato slices and cook for 4 minutes.

Add the cheese and cook for another minute.

Serve warm.

236. Sweet Potatoes and Onions with Jerk Sauce

Preparation Time: 6 Minutes

Servings: 6

Ingredients:

2sweet potatoes, peeled and diced

1pound tempeh, diced

½ sweet onion, diced

¼teaspoon cayenne pepper

1garlic clove, crushed

¼teaspoon paprika

2scallions, coarsely chopped

2teaspoons soy sauce

1tablespoon ginger

2tablespoons lime

1teaspoon dried thyme

1teaspoon dark brown sugar

1hot green chile, seeded and chopped

½teaspoon ground allspice

¼teaspoon ground cinnamon

½teaspoon salt

1tablespoon rice vinegar

¼teaspoon black pepper

⅓cup water

½large or 1 small Vidalia or other sweet onion, cut into ½-inch dice

Directions:

In a blender add the chile, scallions, ginger, garlic and onion.

Blend for 30 seconds and add the soy sauce, cinnamon, cayenne, seasoning, vinegar, marmalade, allspice, sugar and thyme.

Add some water and blend again.

Add the tempeh, onion and potatoes in the instant pot.

Add the jerk sauce you made.

Mix well and cook for 5 minutes.

Serve warm.

237. Ziti Mushroom Stew

 Preparation Time: 6 Minutes

Servings: 4

Ingredients:

1bell pepper, seeded and minced

1onion, minced

1 (14-ouncecan crushed tomatoes

4garlic cloves, minced

2tablespoons tomato paste

½cup dry red wine

8ounces white mushrooms, coarsely chopped

1cup hot water

8ounces uncooked ziti

1teaspoon dried basil

Salt and black pepper

2teaspoons minced fresh oregano

1teaspoon natural sugar

2tablespoons chopped parsley

Directions:

Add the ziti, mushroom, red wine, tomato paste in an instant pot.

Add the sugar, herbs, spices, hot water and the rest of the ingredients.

Mix well and cook for 5 minutes with the lid on.

Serve hot.

Chapter 8.Organic Fruits And Vegetables

238. Baked Potatoes and "BBQ" Lentils

Preparation Time: 5 mins

Servings: 4

Ingredients:

2 sliced large baked potatoes

1 c. dry brown lentils

2 tsps. molasses

1 chopped small onion

2 tsps. liquid smoke

3 c. water

½ c. organic ketchup

Directions:

Add water, onion and lentils to the pot

Lock up the lid and cook on HIGH pressure for 10 minutes

Release the pressure naturally

Add ketchup, liquid smoke and molasses to the lentil

Sauté for 5 minutes

Serve over baked potatoes and enjoy!

Nutrition:

Calories: 140, Fat:4 g, Carbs:24 g, Protein:5 g, Sugars:606 g, Sodium:18 mg

239. Superb Lemon Roasted Artichokes

Preparation Time: 10 mins

Servingss: 2

Ingredients

2 peeled and sliced garlic cloves

3 lemon pieces

Black pepper

2 artichoke pieces

3 tbsps. olive oil

Sea flavored vinegar

Directions:

Wash your artichokes well and dip them in water and cut the stem to about ½ inch long

Trim the thorny tips and outer leaves and rub the chokes with lemon

Poke garlic slivers between the choke leaves and place a trivet basket in the Instant Pot ten add artichokes

Lock up the lid and cook on high pressure for 7 minutes

Release the pressure naturally over 10 minutes

Transfer the artichokes to cutting board and allow them to cool then cut half lengthwise and cut the purple white center

Pre-heat your oven to 400 degree Fahrenheit

Take a bowl and mix 1 and ½ lemon and olive oil

Pour over the choke halves and sprinkle flavored vinegar and pepper

Place an iron skillet in your oven and heat it up for 5 minutes

Add a few teaspoon of oil and place the marinated artichoke halves in the skillet

Brush with lemon and olive oil mixture

Cut third lemon in quarter and nestle them between the halves

Roast for 20-25 minutes until the chokes are browned

Serve and enjoy!

Nutrition:

Calories: 263, Fat:16 g, Carbs:8 g, Protein:23 g, Sugars:128 g, Sodium:0.4 mg

240. Orange Juice Smoothie

Preparation Time: 5 mins

Servingss: 2

Ingredients:

¼ c. frozen orange juice concentrate

¾ c. fat-free milk

1 c. fat-free vanilla frozen yogurt

Directions:

Add the ingredients to a blender and pulse until they're smooth.

Pour them into frosted glasses and serve.

Nutrition:

Calories: 180, Fat:0 g, Carbs:38 g, Protein:7 g, Sugars:20 g, Sodium:5 mg

241. Chocolate Aquafaba Mousse

Preparation Time: 20 mins

Servingss: 4-6

Ingredients:

1 tsp. pure vanilla extract

15 oz. unsalted chickpeas

Fresh raspberries

¼ tsp. tartar cream

6 oz. dairy-free dark chocolate

2 tbsps. coconut sugar

¼ tsp. sea salt

Directions:

Chop dark chocolate into coarse bits and place the chocolate into a glass bowl over boiling water on the stovetop or in a double boiler.

Melt the chocolate gently, stirring until completely melted.

Remove the melted chocolate from the heat and pour the chocolate into a large bowl.

Drain the chickpeas, reserving the brine (aquafaba), and store the chickpeas for another recipe like hummus.

Add in the aquafaba along with cream of tartar.

Mix on high speed using an electric hand mixer for 7-10 minutes, or until soft peaks begin to form.

Add in the salt, vanilla extract, and coconut sugar and beat the mixture until well mixed.

Add half of the melted chocolate to the whipped aquafaba and fold it in until incorporated.

Fold in the remaining aquafaba until smooth and well combined to form the mousse.

Gently spoon the chocolate mousse into glasses, ramekins or small mason jars.

Cover with cling film and chill for at least 3 hours.

Sprinkle he mousse with raspberries and serve.

Nutrition:

Calories: 280, Fat:13.8 g, Carbs:34.7 g, Protein:3.9 g, Sugars:22 g, Sodium:242 mg

242. Minted Peas Feta Rice

Preparation Time: 15 mins

Servingss: 2

Ingredients:

1 ¼ c. vegetable broth

¾ c. brown rice

¼ c. finely crumbled feta cheese

¾ c. sliced scallions

1 ½ c. frozen peas

Freshly ground pepper

¼ c. sliced fresh mint

Directions:

Boil broth in a saucepan over medium heat.

Add rice and bring it to a simmer. Cook for 4 minutes.

Stir in peas and cook for 6 minutes.

Turn off the heat then add feta, mint, scallions, and pepper.

Serve warm.

Nutrition:

Calories: 28.1, Fat:18.2 g, Carbs:10.3 g, Protein:8.8 g, Sugars:2.2 g, Sodium:216 mg

243. Hearty Baby Carrots

Preparation Time: 5 mins

Servingss: 4

Ingredients:

1 tbsp. chopped fresh mint

1 c. water

Sea flavored vinegar

1 lb. baby carrots

1 tbsp. clarified ghee

Directions:

Place a steamer rack on top of your pot and add the carrots

Add water

Lock up the lid and cook at HIGH pressure for 2 minutes

Do a quick release

Pass the carrots through a strainer and drain them

Wipe the insert clean

Return the insert to the pot and set the pot to Sauté mode

Add clarified butter and allow it to melt

Add mint and sauté for 30 seconds

Add carrots to the insert and sauté well

Remove them and sprinkle with bit of flavored vinegar on top

Enjoy!

Nutrition:

Calories: 131, Fat:10 g, Carbs:11 g, Protein:1 g, Sugars:5 g, Sodium:190 mg

244. Sensitive Steamed Artichokes

Preparation Time: 5 mins

Servingss: 4

Ingredients:

1 halved lemon

¼ tsp. paprika

2 tbsps. Homemade Whole30 mayo

2 medium artichokes

1 tsp. Dijon mustard

Directions:

Wash the artichokes and remove the damaged outer leaves

Trim the spines and cut off upper edge

Wipe the cur edges with lemon half

Slice the stem and peel the stem

Chop it up and keep them on the side

Add a cup of water to the pot and place a steamer basket inside

Transfer the artichokes to the steamer basket and a squeeze of lemon

Lock up the lid and cook on HIGH pressure for 10 minutes

Release the pressure naturally

Enjoy

Nutrition:

Calories: 77, Fat:5 g, Carbs:0 g, Protein:2 g, Sugars:1.3 g, Sodium:121 mg

245. Rhubarb and Strawberry Compote

Preparation Time: 10 mins

Servingss: 4

Ingredients:

3 tbsps. Date paste

½ c. water

Fresh mint

2 lbs. rhubarb

1 lb. strawberries

Directions:

Peel the rhubarb using a paring knife and chop it up ½ inch pieces

Add the chopped up rhubarb to your pot alongside water

Lock up the lid and cook on HIGH pressure for 10 minutes

Stem and quarter your strawberries and keep them on the side

Add the strawberries and date paste, give it a nice stir

Lock up the lid and cook on HIGH pressure for 20 minutes

Release the pressure naturally and enjoy the compote!

Nutrition:

Calories: 41.1, Fat:2.1 g, Carbs:5.5 g, Protein:1.4 g, Sugars:12 g, Sodium:2.4 mg

246. Zucchini Cakes

Preparation Time: 10 mins

Servingss: 4

Ingredients:

Freshly ground black pepper

1 finely diced red onion

2 tsps. Salt

1 egg white

Homemade horseradish sauce

1 shredded medium zucchini

¾ c. salt-free bread crumbs

Directions:

Preheat oven to 400°F. Spray a baking sheet lightly with oil and set aside.

Press shredded zucchini gently between paper towels to remove excess liquid.

In a large bowl, combine zucchini, onion, egg white, bread crumbs, seasoning, and black pepper. Mix well.

Shape mixture into patties and place on the prepared baking sheet.

Place baking sheet on middle rack in oven and bake for 10 minutes. Gently flip patties and return to oven to bake for another 10 minutes.

Remove from oven and serve immediately.

Nutrition:

Calories: 94, Fat:1 g, Carbs:19 g, Protein:4 g, Sugars:31 g, Sodium:161 mg

247. Fresh Fruit Smoothie

Preparation Time: 5 mins

Servingss: 4

Ingredients:

1 tbsp. honey

½ c. cantaloupe

1 c. water

1 c. fresh strawberries

1 c. fresh pineapple

2 orange juice

Directions:

Remove the rind from the melon and pineapple. Cut them into chunks and remove the stems from the strawberries.

Put everything in a blender and serve.

Nutrition:

Calories: 72, Fat:1 g, Carbs:17 g, Protein:1 g, Sugars:1 g, Sodium:42 mg

248. Popovers

Preparation Time: 5 mins

Servingss: 6

Ingredients:

4 egg whites

1 c. All-purpose flour

1 c. fat-free milk

¼ tsp. salt

Directions:

Preheat your oven to 425 0F.

Coat a six cup metal or glass muffin mold with cooking spray and heat the mold in the oven for two minutes.

In a bowl, add the flour, milk, salt, and egg whites. Use a mixer to beat until it's smooth.

Fill the heated molds two-thirds of the way full.

Bake until the muffins are golden brown and puffy, around half an hour. Serve.

Nutrition:

Calories: 101, Fat:0 g, Carbs:18 g, Protein:6 g, Sugars:2 g, Sodium:125 mg

249. Broccoli, Garlic, and Rigatoni

Preparation Time: 10 mins

Servings: 2

Ingredients:

2 tsps. Minced garlic

2 c. Broccoli florets

Freshly ground black pepper

2 tbsps. Parmesan cheese

1/3 lb. Rigatoni noodles

2 tsps. Olive oil

Directions:

Fill a pot three-quarters of the way full with water and bring it to a boil. Add the rigatoni and cook until it is firm, around twelve minutes. Drain it thoroughly.

As the pasta cooks, bring an inch of water to a boil and put a steamer basket over the top. Add the broccoli and steam for ten minutes.

In a bowl, mix together the pasta and broccoli. Toss with the cheese, oil, and garlic.

Season to taste and serve.

Nutrition:

Calories: 355, Fat:7 g, Carbs:63 g, Protein:14 g, Sugars:4 g, Sodium:600 mg

250. Vegan Rice Pudding

Preparation Time: 5 mins

Servingss: 8

Ingredients:

½ tsp. ground cinnamon

1 c. rinsed basmati

1/8 tsp. ground cardamom

¼ c. sugar

1/8 tsp. pure almond extract

1 quart vanilla nondairy milk

1 tsp. pure vanilla extract

Directions:

Measure all of the ingredients into a saucepan and stir well to combine. Bring to a boil over medium-high heat.

Once boiling, reduce heat to low and simmer, stirring very frequently, about 15–20 minutes.

Remove from heat and cool. Serve sprinkled with additional ground cinnamon if desired.

Nutrition:

Calories: 148, Fat:2 g, Carbs:26 g, Protein:4 g, Sugars:35 g, Sodium:150 mg

251. Cinnamon-Scented Quinoa

Preparation Time: 5 mins

Servingss: 4

Ingredients:

Chopped walnuts

1 ½ c. water

Maple syrup

2 cinnamon sticks

1 c. quinoa

Directions:

Add the quinoa to a bowl and wash it in several changes of water until the water is clear. When washing quinoa, rub grains and allow them to settle before you pour off the water.

Use a large fine-mesh sieve to drain the quinoa. Prepare your pressure cooker with a trivet and steaming basket. Place the quinoa and the cinnamon sticks in the basket and pour the water.

Close and lock the lid. Cook at high pressure for 6 minutes. When the cooking time is up, release the pressure using the quick release method.

Fluff the quinoa with a fork and remove the cinnamon sticks. Divide the cooked quinoa among serving bowls and top with maple syrup and chopped walnuts.

Nutrition:

Calories: 160, Fat:3 g, Carbs:28 g, Protein:6 g, Sugars:19 g, Sodium:40 mg

252. Green Vegetable Smoothie

Preparation Time: 5 mins

Servingss: 4

Ingredients:

1 c. cold water

½ c. strawberries

2 oz. baby spinach

1 lemon juice

1 tbsp. fresh mint

1 banana

½ c. blueberries

Directions:

Put all the ingredients in a juicer or blender and puree.

Nutrition:

Calories: 52, Fat:2 g, Carbs:12 g, Protein:1 g, Sugars:18 g, Sodium:36 mg

253. Garlic Lovers Hummus

Preparation Time: 2 mins

Servingss: 12

Ingredients:

3 tbsps. Freshly squeezed lemon juice

All-purpose salt-free seasoning

3 tbsps. Sesame tahini

4 garlic cloves

15 oz. no-salt-added garbanzo beans

2 tbsps. Olive oil

Directions:

Drain garbanzo beans and rinse well.

Place all the ingredients in a food processor and pulse until smooth.

Serve immediately or cover and refrigerate until serving.

Nutrition:

Calories: 103, Fat:5 g, Carbs:11 g, Protein:4 g, Sugars:2 g, Sodium:88 mg

254. Spinach and Kale Mix

Preparation Time: 5 mins

Servingss: 4

Ingredients:

2 chopped shallots

1 c. no-salt-added and chopped canned tomatoes

2 c. baby spinach

2 minced garlic cloves

5 c. torn kale

1 tbsp. olive oil

Directions:

Heat up a pan with the oil over medium-high heat, add the shallots, stir and sauté for 5 minutes.

Add the spinach, kale and the other ingredients, toss, cook for 10 minutes more, divide between plates and serve.

Nutrition:

Calories: 89, Fat:3.7 g, Carbs:12.4 g, Protein:3.6 g, Sugars:0 g, Sodium:50 mg

255. Apples and Cabbage Mix

Preparation Time: 5 mins

Servingss: 4

Ingredients:

2 cored and cubed green apples

2 tbsps. balsamic vinegar

½ tsp. caraway seeds

2 tbsps. olive oil

Black pepper

1 shredded red cabbage head

Directions:

In a bowl, combine the cabbage with the apples and the other ingredients, toss and serve.

Nutrition:

Calories: 165, Fat:7.4 g, Carbs:26 g, Protein:2.6 g, Sugars:2.6 g, Sodium:19 mg

256. Thyme Mushrooms

Preparation Time: 10 mins

Servingss: 4

Ingredients:

1 tbsp. chopped thyme

2 tbsps. olive oil

2 tbsps. chopped parsley

4 minced garlic cloves

Black pepper

2 lbs. halved white mushrooms

Directions:

In a baking pan, combine the mushrooms with the garlic and the other ingredients, toss, introduce in the oven and cook at 400 0F for 30 minutes.

Divide between plates and serve.

Nutrition:

Calories: 251, Fat:9.3 g, Carbs:13.2 g, Protein:6 g, Sugars:0.8 g, Sodium:37 mg

257. Rosemary Endives

Preparation Time: 10 mins

Servingss: 4

Ingredients:

2 tbsps. olive oil

1 tsp. dried rosemary

2 halved endives

¼ tsp. black pepper

½ tsp. turmeric powder

Directions:

In a baking pan, combine the endives with the oil and the other ingredients, toss gently, introduce in the oven and bake at 400 0F for 20 minutes.

Divide between plates and serve.

Nutrition:

Calories: 66, Fat:7.1 g, Carbs:1.2 g, Protein:0.3 g, Sugars:1.3 g, Sodium:113 mg

258. Kale Sauté

Preparation Time: 10 mins

Servingss: 4

Ingredients:

1 chopped red onion

3 tbsps. coconut aminos

2 tbsps. olive oil

1 lb. torn kale

1 tbsp. chopped cilantro

1 tbsp. lime juice

2 minced garlic cloves

Directions:

Heat up a pan with the olive oil over medium heat, add the onion and the garlic and sauté for 5 minutes.

Add the kale and the other ingredients, toss, cook over medium heat for 10 minutes, divide between plates and serve.

Nutrition:

Calories: 200, Fat:7.1 g, Carbs:6.4 g, Protein:6 g, Sugars:1.6 g, Sodium:183 mg

259. Roasted Beets

Preparation Time: 10 mins

Servingss: 4

Ingredients:

2 minced garlic cloves

¼ tsp. black pepper

4 peeled and sliced beets

¼ c. chopped walnuts

2 tbsps. olive oil

¼ c. chopped parsley

Directions:

In a baking dish, combine the beets with the oil and the other ingredients, toss to coat, introduce in the oven at 420 0F, and bake for 30 minutes.

Divide between plates and serve.

Nutrition:

Calories: 156, Fat:11.8 g, Carbs:11.5 g, Protein:3.8 g, Sugars:8 g, Sodium:670 mg

260. Minty Tomatoes and Corn

Preparation Time: 5 mins

Servingss: 4

Ingredients:

2 c. corn

1 tbsp. rosemary vinegar

2 tbsps. chopped mint

1 lb. sliced tomatoes

¼ tsp. black pepper

2 tbsps. olive oil

Directions:

In a salad bowl, combine the tomatoes with the corn and the other ingredients, toss and serve.

Enjoy!

Nutrition:

Calories: 230, Fat:7.2 g, Carbs:11.6 g, Protein:4 g, Sugars:1 g, Sodium:53 mg

261. Pesto Green Beans

Preparation Time: 10 mins

Servingss: 4

Ingredients:

2 tbsps. olive oil

2 tsps. sweet paprika

Juice of 1 lemon

2 tbsps. basil pesto

1 lb. trimmed and halved green beans

¼ tsp. black pepper

1 sliced red onion

Directions:

Heat up a pan with the oil over medium-high heat, add the onion, stir and sauté for 5 minutes.

Add the beans and the rest of the ingredients, toss, cook over medium heat for 10 minutes, divide between plates and serve.

Nutrition:

Calories: 280, Fat:10 g, Carbs:13.9 g, Protein:4.7 g, Sugars:0.8 g, Sodium:138 mg

262. Sage Carrots

Preparation Time: 10 mins

Servingss: 4

Ingredients:

2 tsps. sweet paprika

1 tbsp. chopped sage

2 tbsps. olive oil

1 lb. peeled and roughly cubed carrots

¼ tsp. black pepper

1 chopped red onion

Directions:

In a baking pan, combine the carrots with the oil and the other ingredients, toss and bake at 380 0F for 30 minutes.

Divide between plates and serve.

Nutrition:

Calories: 200, Fat:8.7 g, Carbs:7.9 g, Protein:4 g, Sugars:19 g, Sodium:268 mg

263. Dates and Cabbage Sauté

Preparation Time: 5 mins

Servingss: 4

Ingredients:

2 tbsps. olive oil

2 tbsps. lemon juice

1 lb. shredded red cabbage

Black pepper

8 pitted and sliced dates

2 tbsps. chopped chives

¼ c. low-sodium veggie stock

Directions:

Heat up a pan with the oil over medium heat, add the cabbage and the dates, toss and cook for 4 minutes.

Add the stock and the other ingredients, toss, cook over medium heat for 11 minutes more, divide between plates and serve.

Nutrition:

Calories: 280, Fat:8.1 g, Carbs:8.7 g, Protein:6.3 g, Sugars:4.7 g, Sodium:430 mg

264. Baked Squash Mix

Preparation Time: 10 mins

Servingss: 4

Ingredients:

2 tsps. chopped cilantro

2 lbs. peeled and sliced butternut squash

¼ tsp. black pepper

1 tsp. garlic powder

2 tbsps. olive oil

1 tsp. chili powder

1 tbsp. lemon juice

Directions:

In a roasting pan, combine the squash with the oil and the other ingredients, toss gently, bake in the oven at 400 0F for 45 minutes, divide between plates and serve.

Nutrition:

Calories: 167, Fat:7.4 g, Carbs:27.5 g, Protein:2.5 g, Sugars:4.4 g, Sodium:10 mg

265. Lemony Endives

Preparation Time: 10 mins

Servingss: 4

Ingredients:

1 tbsps. grated lemon zest

4 halved endives

2 tbsps. olive oil

1 tbsp. lemon juice

¼ tsp. black pepper

2 tbsps. grated fat-free parmesan

Directions:

In a baking dish, combine the endives with the lemon juice and the other ingredients except the parmesan and toss.

Sprinkle the parmesan on top, bake the endives at 400 0F for 20 minutes, divide between plates and serve as a side dish.

Nutrition:

Calories: 71, Fat:7.1 g, Carbs:2.3 g, Protein:0.9 g, Sugars:2 g, Sodium:58 mg

266. Garlic Mushrooms and Corn

Preparation Time: 10 mins

Servingss: 4

Ingredients:

2 c. corn

1 lb. halved white mushrooms

¼ tsp. black pepper

½ tsp. chili powder

2 tbsps. olive oil

1 c. no-salt-added, chopped and canned tomatoes

4 minced garlic cloves

Directions:

Heat up a pan with the oil over medium heat, add the mushrooms, garlic and the corn, stir and sauté for 10 minutes.

Add the rest of the ingredients, toss, cook over medium heat for 10 minutes more, divide between plates and serve.

Nutrition:

Calories: 285, Fat:13 g, Carbs:14.6 g, Protein:6.7 g, Sugars:2 g, Sodium:260 mg

267. Cilantro Broccoli

Preparation Time: 10 mins

Servingss: 4

Ingredients:

2 tbsps. chili sauce

2 tbsps. olive oil

2 minced garlic cloves

¼ tsp. black pepper

1 lb. broccoli florets

2 tbsps. chopped cilantro

1 tbsp. lemon juice

Directions:

In a baking pan, combine the broccoli with the oil, garlic and the other ingredients, toss a bit, introduce in the oven and bake at 400 0F for 30 minutes.

Divide the mix between plates and serve.

Nutrition:

Calories: 103, Fat:7.4 g, Carbs:8.3 g, Protein:3.4 g, Sugars:33 g, Sodium:1.7 mg

268. Paprika Carrots

Preparation Time: 10 mins

Servingss: 4

Ingredients:

1 tbsp. sweet paprika

1 tsp. lime juice

1 lb. trimmed baby carrots

¼ tsp. black pepper

3 tbsps. olive oil

1 tsp. sesame seeds

Directions:

Arrange the carrots on a lined baking sheet, add the paprika and the other ingredients except the sesame seeds, toss, introduce in the oven and bake at 400 0F for 30 minutes.

Divide the carrots between plates, sprinkle sesame seeds on top and serve.

Nutrition:

Calories: 142, Fat:11.3 g, Carbs:11.4 g, Protein:1.2 g, Sugars:7 g, Sodium:200 mg

269. Mashed Cauliflower

Preparation Time: 10 mins

Servingss: 4

Ingredients:

½ c. coconut milk

1 tbsp. chopped chives

2 lbs. cauliflower florets

¼ tsp. black pepper

1 tbsp. chopped cilantro

½ c. low-fat sour cream

Directions:

Put the cauliflower in a pot, add water to cover, bring to a boil over medium heat, and cook for 25 minutes and drain.

Mash the cauliflower, add the milk, black pepper and the cream, whisk well, divide between plates, sprinkle the rest of the ingredients on top and serve.

Nutrition:

Calories: 188, Fat:13.4 g, Carbs:15 g, Protein:6.1 g, Sugars:5 g, Sodium:339 mg

270. Spinach Spread

Preparation Time: 10 mins

Servingss: 4

Ingredients:

1 c. coconut cream

1 tbsp. chopped dill

1 lb. chopped spinach

¼ tsp. black pepper

1 c. shredded low-fat mozzarella

Directions:

In a baking pan, combine the spinach with the cream and the other ingredients, stir well, introduce in the oven and bake at 400 0F for 20 minutes.

Divide into bowls and serve.

Nutrition:

Calories: 340, Fat:33 g, Carbs:4 g, Protein:5 g, Sugars:3 g, Sodium:640 mg

271. Mustard Greens Sauté

Preparation Time: 10 mins

Servingss: 4

Ingredients:

2 tbsps. olive oil

2 chopped spring onions

6 c. mustard greens

2 tbsps. sweet paprika

Black pepper

½ c. coconut cream

Directions:

Heat up a pan with the oil over medium-high heat, add the onions, paprika and black pepper, stir and sauté for 3 minutes.

Add the mustard greens and the other ingredients, toss, cook for 9 minutes more, divide between plates and serve.

Nutrition:

Calories: 163, Fat:14.8 g, Carbs:8.3 g, Protein:3.6 g, Sugars:7 g, Sodium:390 mg

272. Basil Turnips Mix

Preparation Time: 10 mins

Servingss: 4

Ingredients:

¼ c. low-sodium veggie stock

4 sliced turnips

¼ c. chopped basil

2 minced garlic cloves

1 tbsp. avocado oil

½ c. chopped walnuts

Black pepper

Directions:

Heat up a pan with the oil over medium-high heat, add the garlic and the turnips and brown for 5 minutes.

Add the rest of the ingredients, toss, cook for 10 minutes more, divide between plates and serve.

Nutrition:

Calories: 140, Fat:9.7 g, Carbs:10.5 g, Protein:5 g, Sugars:3 g, Sodium:357 mg

273. Baked Mushrooms

Preparation Time: 10 mins

Servingss: 4

Ingredients:

Black pepper

1 tbsp. chopped chives

1 lb. small mushroom caps

1 tbsp. chopped rosemary

2 tbsps. olive oil

Directions:

Put the mushrooms in a roasting pan, add the oil and the rest of the ingredients, toss, bake at 400 0F for 25 minutes, divide into bowls and serve

Nutrition:

Calories: 215, Fat:12.3 g, Carbs:15.3 g, Protein:3.5 g, Sugars:4.5 g, Sodium:309 mg

274. Celery and Kale Mix

Preparation Time: 10 mins

Servingss: 4

Ingredients:

5 c. torn kale

2 chopped celery stalks

1 tbsp. extra-virgin olive oil

3 tbsps. water

Directions:

Heat up a pan while using the oil over medium-high heat, add celery, stir and cook for 10 minutes.

Add kale and water, toss, cook for ten minutes more, divide between plates and serve.

Enjoy!

Nutrition:

Calories: 140, Fat:1 g, Carbs:6 g, Protein:6 g, Sugars:20 g, Sodium:169 mg

275. Spicy Avocado

Preparation Time: 10 mins

Servingss: 1

Ingredients:

2 tbsps. hot sauce

Sea salt

1 c. halved ripe avocado

½ Juiced lemon

Directions:

Slice the avocado in half a few times, spin and slice a few more times perpendicular to the first slices. You should end up with several cubes that are still attached to the peel.

Drizzle the lemon juice and hot sauce onto the avocado. Eat with a fork.

Nutrition:

Calories: 124, Fat:10.8 g, Carbs:9.5 g, Protein:1.9 g, Sugars:0.4 g, Sodium:95 mg

276. Cauliflower Risotto

Preparation Time: 10 mins

Servingss: 4

Ingredients:

2 minced garlic cloves

1 tbsp. fresh lemon juice

2 tbsps. essential organic olive oil

2 tbsps. chopped thyme

¼ tsp. black pepper

12 oz. cauliflower rice

Zest of ½ grated lemon

Directions:

Heat up a pan with the oil over medium-high heat, add cauliflower rice and garlic, stir and cook for 5 minutes.

Add freshly squeezed fresh lemon juice, lemon zest, thyme, salt and pepper, stir, cook for two main minutes more, divide between plates and serve.

Enjoy!

Nutrition:

Calories: 130, Fat:2 g, Carbs:6 g, Protein:8 g, Sugars:0.3 g, Sodium: 160 mg

277. Kale Dip

Preparation Time: 10 mins

Servingss: 4

Ingredients:

1 c. coconut cream

1 tsp. chili powder

1 bunch kale leaves

1 chopped shallot

¼ tsp. black pepper

1 tbsp. olive oil

Directions:

Heat up a pan with the oil over medium heat, add the shallots, stir and sauté for 4 minutes.

Add the kale and the other ingredients, bring to a simmer and cook over medium heat for 16 minutes.

Blend using an immersion blender, divide into bowls and serve.

Nutrition:

Calories: 188, Fat:17.9 g, Carbs:7.6 g, Protein:2.5 g, Sugars:0.8 g, Sodium:23 mg

278. Dill Cabbage

Preparation Time: 10 mins

Servingss: 4

Ingredients:

1 chopped yellow onion

¼ tsp. black pepper

1 lb. shredded green cabbage

1 tbsp. chopped dill

1 tbsp. olive oil

1 cubed tomato

Directions:

Heat up a pan with the oil over medium heat, add the onion and sauté for 5 minutes.

Add the cabbage and the rest of the ingredients, toss, cook over medium heat for 10 minutes, divide between plates and serve.

Nutrition:

Calories: 74, Fat:3.7 g, Carbs:10.2 g, Protein:2.1 g, Sugars:2 g, Sodium:115 mg

279. Curried Cauliflower Steaks with Red Rice

Preparation Time: 6 mins

Servingss: 4

Ingredients:

1/3 c. extra-virgin olive oil

2 tsps. curry powder

½ tsps. kosher salt

2 cauliflower heads

1 tbsp. lemon juice

2 tbsps. chopped fresh cilantro

1 c. brown rice

Directions:

Preheat oven to 450 0F. Line a large baking sheet with tin foil.

Follow directions to prepare rice.

Whisk together oil, curry powder, and salt in a bowl.

Prepare cauliflower, making sure to keep stems intact. Place stem-side down on a cutting board and cut into thick slices to create "steaks." Get 4 steaks. Then slice the remaining cauliflower into smaller slices to get 4 cups.

Place steaks and florets onto a baking sheet. Brush both sides of the steaks with the curry mixture.

Place steaks in oven, turning after 15 minutes. Finish baking until steaks are tender and brown.

Divide rice evenly onto 4 plates and top each plate with a cauliflower steak. Sprinkle with cilantro.

Nutrition:

Calories: 410, Fat:21 g, Carbs:49 g, Protein:10 g, Sugars:5 g, Sodium:317 mg

Chapter 9. Drinks

280. Spiced Buttermilk

Preparation time: 5 minutes

Cooking time: 0 minute

Servings: 2

Ingredients:

3/4 teaspoon ground cumin

1/4 teaspoon sea salt

1/8 teaspoon ground black pepper

2 mint leaves

1/8 teaspoon lemon juice

¼ cup cilantro leaves

1 cup of chilled water

1 cup vegan yogurt, unsweetened

Ice as needed

Directions:

Place all the ingredients in the order in a food processor or blender, except for cilantro and ¼ teaspoon cumin, and then pulse for 2 to 3 minutes at high speed until smooth.

Pour the milk into glasses, top with cilantro and cumin, and then serve.

Nutrition:

Calories: 92 Cal

Fat: 2 g

Carbs: 5 g

Protein: 11 g

Fiber: 0.5 g

281. Turmeric Lassi

Preparation time: 5 minutes

Cooking time: 0 minute

Servings: 2

Ingredients:

1 teaspoon grated ginger

1/8 teaspoon ground black pepper

1 teaspoon turmeric powder

1/8 teaspoon cayenne

1 tablespoon coconut sugar

1/8 teaspoon salt

1 cup vegan yogurt

1 cup almond milk

Directions:

Place all the ingredients in the order in a food processor or blender and then pulse for 2 to 3 minutes at high speed until smooth.

Pour the lassi into two glasses and then serve.

Nutrition:

Calories: 128 Cal

Fat: 3 g

Carbs: 20 g

Protein: 3 g

Fiber: 1 g

282. Brownie Batter Orange Chia Shake

Preparation time: 5 minutes

Cooking time: 0 minute

Servings: 2

Ingredients:

2 tablespoons cocoa powder

3 tablespoons chia seeds

¼ teaspoon salt

4 tablespoons chocolate chips

4 teaspoons coconut sugar

½ teaspoon orange zest

½ teaspoon vanilla extract, unsweetened

2 cup almond milk

Directions:

Place all the ingredients in the order in a food processor or blender and then pulse for 2 to 3 minutes at high speed until smooth.

Pour the smoothie into two glasses and then serve.

Nutrition:

Calories: 487 Cal

Fat: 31 g

Carbs: 57 g

Protein: 9 g

Fiber: 11 g

283. Saffron Pistachio Beverage

Preparation time: 5 minutes

Cooking time: 0 minute

Servings: 2

Ingredients:

8 strands of saffron

1 tablespoon cashews

1/4 teaspoon ground ginger

2 tablespoons pistachio

1/8 teaspoon cloves

1/4 teaspoon ground black pepper

1/4 teaspoon cardamom powder

3 tablespoons coconut sugar

1/4 teaspoon cinnamon

1/8 teaspoon fennel seeds

1/4 teaspoon poppy seeds

Directions:

Place all the ingredients in the order in a food processor or blender and then pulse for 2 to 3 minutes at high speed until smooth.

Pour the smoothie into two glasses and then serve.

Nutrition:

Calories: 96 Cal

Fat: 3 g

Carbs: 15 g

Protein: 1 g

Fiber: 3 g

284. Mexican Hot Chocolate Mix

Preparation time: 5 minutes

Cooking time: 0 minute

Servings: 2

Ingredients:

For the Hot Chocolate Mix:

1/3 cup chopped dark chocolate

1/8 teaspoon cayenne

1/8 teaspoon salt

1/2 teaspoon cinnamon

1/4 cup coconut sugar

1 teaspoon cornstarch

3 tablespoons cocoa powder

1/2 teaspoon vanilla extract, unsweetened

For Serving:

2 cups milk, warmed

Directions:

Place all the ingredients of hot chocolate mix in the order in a food processor or blender and then pulse for 2 to 3 minutes at high speed until ground.

Stir 2 tablespoons of the chocolate mix into a glass of milk until combined and then serve.

Nutrition:

Calories: 127 Cal

Fat: 5 g

Carbs: 20 g

Protein: 1 g

Fiber: 2 g

285. Pumpkin Spice Frappuccino

Preparation time: 5 minutes

Cooking time: 0 minute

Servings: 2

Ingredients:

½ teaspoon ground ginger

1/8 teaspoon allspice

½ teaspoon ground cinnamon

2 tablespoons coconut sugar

1/8 teaspoon nutmeg

¼ teaspoon ground cloves

1 teaspoon vanilla extract, unsweetened

2 teaspoons instant coffee

2 cups almond milk, unsweetened

1 cup of ice cubes

Directions:

Place all the ingredients in the order in a food processor or blender and then pulse for 2 to 3 minutes at high speed until smooth.

Pour the Frappuccino into two glasses and then serve.

Nutrition:

Calories: 90 Cal

Fat: 6 g

Carbs: 5 g

Protein: 2 g

Fiber: 1 g

286. Cookie Dough Milkshake

Preparation time: 5 minutes

Cooking time: 0 minute

Servings: 2

Ingredients:

2 tablespoons cookie dough

5 dates, pitted

2 teaspoons chocolate chips

1/2 teaspoon vanilla extract, unsweetened

1/2 cup almond milk, unsweetened

1 ½ cup almond milk ice cubes

Directions:

Place all the ingredients in the order in a food processor or blender and then pulse for 2 to 3 minutes at high speed until smooth.

Pour the milkshake into two glasses and then serve with some cookie dough balls.

Nutrition:

Calories: 208 Cal

Fat: 9 g

Carbs: 30 g

Protein: 2 g

Fiber: 2 g

287. Strawberry and Hemp Smoothie

Preparation time: 5 minutes

Cooking time: 0 minute

Servings: 2

Ingredients:

3 cups fresh strawberries

2 tablespoons hemp seeds

1/2 teaspoon vanilla extract, unsweetened

1/8 teaspoon sea salt

2 tablespoons maple syrup

1 cup vegan yogurt

1 cup almond milk, unsweetened

1 cup of ice cubes

2 tablespoons hemp protein

Directions:

Place all the ingredients in the order in a food processor or blender, except for protein powder, and then pulse for 2 to 3 minutes at high speed until smooth.

Pour the smoothie into two glasses and then serve.

Nutrition:

Calories: 258 Cal

Fat: 17 g

Carbs: 12 g

Protein: 14 g

Fiber: 2 g

288. Blueberry, Hazelnut and Hemp Smoothie

Preparation time: 5 minutes

Cooking time: 0 minute

Servings: 2

Ingredients:

2 tablespoons hemp seeds

1 ½ cups frozen blueberries

2 tablespoons chocolate protein powder

1/2 teaspoon vanilla extract, unsweetened

2 tablespoons chocolate hazelnut butter

1 small frozen banana

3/4 cup almond milk

Directions:

Place all the ingredients in the order in a food processor or blender and then pulse for 2 to 3 minutes at high speed until smooth.

Pour the smoothie into two glasses and then serve.

Nutrition:

Calories: 376 Cal

Fat: 25 g

Carbs: 26 g

Protein: 14 g

Fiber: 4 g

289. Mango Lassi

Preparation time: 5 minutes

Cooking time: 0 minute

Servings: 2

Ingredients:

1 ¼ cup mango pulp

1 tablespoon coconut sugar

1/8 teaspoon salt

1/2 teaspoon lemon juice

1/4 cup almond milk, unsweetened

1/4 cup chilled water

1 cup cashew yogurt

Directions:

Place all the ingredients in the order in a food processor or blender and then pulse for 2 to 3 minutes at high speed until smooth.

Pour the lassi into two glasses and then serve.

Nutrition:

Calories: 218 Cal

Fat: 2 g

Carbs: 44 g

Protein: 3 g

Fiber: 1 g

290. Mocha Chocolate Shake

Preparation time: 5 minutes

Cooking time: 0 minute

Servings: 2

Ingredients:

1/4 cup hemp seeds

2 teaspoons cocoa powder, unsweetened

1/2 cup dates, pitted

1 tablespoon instant coffee powder

2 tablespoons flax seeds

2 1/2 cups almond milk, unsweetened

1/2 cup crushed ice

Directions:

Place all the ingredients in the order in a food processor or blender and then pulse for 2 to 3 minutes at high speed until smooth.

Pour the smoothie into two glasses and then serve.

Nutrition:

Calories: 357 Cal

Fat: 21 g

Carbs: 31 g

Protein: 12 g

Fiber: 5 g

291. Chard, Lettuce and Ginger Smoothie

Preparation time: 5 minutes

Cooking time: 0 minute

Servings: 2

Ingredients:

10 Chard leaves, chopped

1-inch piece of ginger, chopped

10 lettuce leaves, chopped

½ teaspoon black salt

2 pear, chopped

2 teaspoons coconut sugar

¼ teaspoon ground black pepper

¼ teaspoon salt

2 tablespoons lemon juice

2 cups of water

Directions:

Place all the ingredients in the order in a food processor or blender and then pulse for 2 to 3 minutes at high speed until smooth.

Pour the smoothie into two glasses and then serve.

Nutrition:

Calories: 514 Cal

Fat: 0 g

Carbs: 15 g

Protein: 4 g

Fiber: 4 g

292. Red Beet, Pear and Apple Smoothie

Preparation time: 5 minutes

Cooking time: 0 minute

Servings: 2

Ingredients:

1/2 of medium beet, peeled, chopped

1 tablespoon chopped cilantro

1 orange, juiced

1 medium pear, chopped

1 medium apple, cored, chopped

1/4 teaspoon ground black pepper

1/8 teaspoon rock salt

1 teaspoon coconut sugar

1/4 teaspoons salt

1 cup of water

Directions:

Place all the ingredients in the order in a food processor or blender and then pulse for 2 to 3 minutes at high speed until smooth.

Pour the smoothie into two glasses and then serve.

Nutrition:

Calories: 132 Cal

Fat: 0 g

Carbs: 34 g

Protein: 1 g

Fiber: 5 g

293. Berry and Yogurt Smoothie

Preparation time: 5 minutes

Cooking time: 0 minute

Servings: 2

Ingredients:

2 small bananas

3 cups frozen mixed berries

1 ½ cup cashew yogurt

1/2 teaspoon vanilla extract, unsweetened

1/2 cup almond milk, unsweetened

Directions:

Place all the ingredients in the order in a food processor or blender and then pulse for 2 to 3 minutes at high speed until smooth.

Pour the smoothie into two glasses and then serve.

Nutrition:

Calories: 326 Cal

Fat: 6.5 g

Carbs: 65.6 g

Protein: 8 g

Fiber: 8.4 g

294. Chocolate and Cherry Smoothie

Preparation time: 5 minutes

Cooking time: 0 minute

Servings: 2

Ingredients:

4 cups frozen cherries

2 tablespoons cocoa powder

1 scoop of protein powder

1 teaspoon maple syrup

2 cups almond milk, unsweetened

Directions:

Place all the ingredients in the order in a food processor or blender and then pulse for 2 to 3 minutes at high speed until smooth.

Pour the smoothie into two glasses and then serve.

Nutrition:

Calories: 324 Cal

Fat: 5 g

Carbs: 75.1 g

Protein: 7.2 g

Fiber: 11.3 g

295. Strawberry and Chocolate Milkshake

Preparation time: 5 minutes

Cooking time: 0 minute

Servings: 2

Ingredients:

2 cups frozen strawberries

3 tablespoons cocoa powder

1 scoop protein powder

2 tablespoons maple syrup

1 teaspoon vanilla extract, unsweetened

2 cups almond milk, unsweetened

Directions:

Place all the ingredients in the order in a food processor or blender and then pulse for 2 to 3 minutes at high speed until smooth.

Pour the smoothie into two glasses and then serve.

Nutrition:

Calories: 199 Cal

Fat: 4.1 g

Carbs: 40.5 g

Protein: 3.7 g

Fiber: 5.5 g

296. Banana and Protein Smoothie

Preparation time: 5 minutes

Cooking time: 0 minute

Servings: 2

Ingredients:

2/3 cup frozen pineapple chunk

10 frozen strawberries

2 frozen bananas

2 scoops protein powder

2 teaspoons cocoa powder

2 tablespoons maple syrup

2 teaspoons vanilla extract, unsweetened

2 cups almond milk, unsweetened

Directions:

Place all the ingredients in the order in a food processor or blender and then pulse for 2 to 3 minutes at high speed until smooth.

Pour the smoothie into two glasses and then serve.

Nutrition:

Calories: 272 Cal

Fat: 3.8 g

Carbs: 59.4 g

Protein: 4.3 g

Fiber: 7.1 g

297. Mango, Pineapple and Banana Smoothie

Preparation time: 5 minutes

Cooking time: 0 minute

Servings: 2

Ingredients:

2 cups pineapple chunks

2 frozen bananas

2 medium mangoes, destoned, cut into chunks

1 cup almond milk, unsweetened

Chia seeds as needed for garnishing

Directions:

Place all the ingredients in the order in a food processor or blender and then pulse for 2 to 3 minutes at high speed until smooth.

Pour the smoothie into two glasses and then serve.

Nutrition:

Calories: 287 Cal

Fat: 1.2 g

Carbs: 73.3 g

Protein: 3.5 g

Fiber: 8 g

298. Blueberry and Banana Smoothie

Preparation time: 5 minutes

Cooking time: 0 minute

Servings: 2

Ingredients:

2 frozen bananas

2 cups frozen blueberries

2 cups almond milk, unsweetened

1/2 teaspoon or so cinnamon

dash of vanilla extract

Directions:

Place all the ingredients in the order in a food processor or blender and then pulse for 2 to 3 minutes at high speed until smooth.

Pour the smoothie into two glasses and then serve.

Nutrition:

Calories: 244 Cal

Fat: 3.8 g

Carbs: 51.5 g

Protein: 4 g

Fiber: 7.3 g

299. 'Sweet Tang' and Chia Smoothie

Preparation time: 5 minutes

Cooking time: 0 minute

Servings: 2

Ingredients:

4 large plums

2 tablespoon chia seeds

1/2 cup pineapple chunks

1/2 cup ice cubes

3/4 cup coconut water

Directions:

Place all the ingredients in the order in a food processor or blender and then pulse for 2 to 3 minutes at high speed until smooth.

Pour the smoothie into two glasses and then serve.

Nutrition:

Calories: 406 Cal

Fat: 9.3 g

Carbs: 77.4 g

Protein: 6.3 g

Fiber: 13 g

300. Strawberry, Mango and Banana Smoothie

Preparation time: 5 minutes

Cooking time: 0 minute

Servings: 2

Ingredients:

1 medium frozen banana

1 cup of frozen strawberries

2 tablespoons ground chia seeds

1 cup chopped mango

2 tablespoons cashew butter

1 cup coconut milk, unsweetened

Directions:

Place all the ingredients in the order in a food processor or blender and then pulse for 2 to 3 minutes at high speed until smooth.

Pour the smoothie into two glasses and then serve.

Nutrition:

Calories: 299 Cal

Fat: 15 g

Carbs: 42 g

Protein: 5 g

Fiber: 8 g

301. Strawberry and Pineapple Smoothie

Preparation time: 5 minutes

Cooking time: 0 minute

Servings: 2

Ingredients:

2 cups frozen strawberries

2 tablespoons almond butter

2 cups chopped pineapple

1 ½ cup chilled almond milk, unsweetened

Directions:

Place all the ingredients in the order in a food processor or blender and then pulse for 2 to 3 minutes at high speed until smooth.

Pour the smoothie into two glasses and then serve.

Nutrition:

Calories: 255 Cal

Fat: 11 g

Carbs: 39 g

Protein: 6 g

Fiber: 8 g

302. Strawberry, Blueberry and Banana Smoothie

Preparation time: 5 minutes

Cooking time: 0 minute

Servings: 2

Ingredients:

1 tablespoon hulled hemp seeds

½ cup of frozen strawberries

1 small frozen banana

½ cup frozen blueberries

2 tablespoons cashew butter

¾ cup cashew milk, unsweetened

Directions:

Place all the ingredients in the order in a food processor or blender and then pulse for 2 to 3 minutes at high speed until smooth.

Pour the smoothie into two glasses and then serve.

Nutrition:

Calories: 334 Cal

Fat: 17 g

Carbs: 46 g

Protein: 7 g

Fiber: 7 g

303. Pineapple and Spinach Juice

Preparation time: 5 minutes

Cooking time: 0 minute

Servings: 2

Ingredients:

2 medium red apples, cored, peeled, chopped

3 cups spinach

½ of a medium pineapple, peeled

2 lemons, peeled

Directions:

Process all the ingredients in the order in a juicer or blender and then strain it into two glasses.

Serve straight away.

Nutrition:

Calories: 131 Cal

Fat: 0.5 g

Carbs: 34.5 g

Protein: 1.7 g

Fiber: 5 g

304. Green Lemonade

Preparation time: 5 minutes

Cooking time: 0 minute

Servings: 2

Ingredients:

10 large stalks of celery, chopped

2 medium green apples, cored, peeled, chopped

2 medium cucumbers, peeled, chopped

2 inches piece of ginger

10 stalks of kale, chopped

2 cups parsley

Directions:

Process all the ingredients in the order in a juicer or blender and then strain it into two glasses.

Serve straight away.

Nutrition:

Calories: 102.3 Cal

Fat: 1.1 g

Carbs: 26.2 g

Protein: 4.7 g

Fiber: 8.5 g

305. Sweet and Sour Juice

Preparation time: 5 minutes

Cooking time: 0 minute

Servings: 2

Ingredients:

2 medium apples, cored, peeled, chopped

2 large cucumbers, peeled

4 cups chopped grapefruit

1 cup mint

Directions:

Process all the ingredients in the order in a juicer or blender and then strain it into two glasses.

Serve straight away.

Nutrition:

Calories: 90 Cal

Fat: 0 g

Carbs: 23 g

Protein: 0 g

Fiber: 9 g

306. Apple, Carrot, Celery and Kale Juice

Preparation time: 5 minutes

Cooking time: 0 minute

Servings: 2

Ingredients:

5 curly kale

2 green apples, cored, peeled, chopped

2 large stalks celery

4 large carrots, cored, peeled, chopped

Directions:

Process all the ingredients in the order in a juicer or blender and then strain it into two glasses.

Serve straight away.

Nutrition:

Calories: 183 Cal

Fat: 2.5 g

Carbs: 46 g

Protein: 13 g

Fiber: 3 g

307. Banana Milk

Preparation time: 5 minutes

Cooking time: 0 minute

Servings: 2

Ingredients:

2 dates

2 medium bananas, peeled

1 teaspoon vanilla extract, unsweetened

1/2 cup ice

2 cups of water

Directions:

Place all the ingredients in the order in a food processor or blender and then pulse for 2 to 3 minutes at high speed until smooth.

Pour the smoothie into two glasses and then serve.

Nutrition:

Calories: 79 Cal

Fat: 0 g

Carbs: 19.8 g

Protein: 0.8 g

Fiber: 6 g

308. Hazelnut and Chocolate Milk

Preparation time: 5 minutes

Cooking time: 0 minute

Servings: 2

Ingredients:

2 tablespoons cocoa powder

4 dates, pitted

1 cup hazelnuts

3 cups of water

Directions:

Place all the ingredients in the order in a food processor or blender and then pulse for 2 to 3 minutes at high speed until smooth.

Pour the smoothie into two glasses and then serve.

Nutrition:

Calories: 120 Cal

Fat: 5 g

Carbs: 19 g

Protein: 2 g

Fiber: 1 g

309. Fruit Infused Water

Preparation time: 5 minutes

Cooking time: 0 minute

Servings: 2

Ingredients:

3 strawberries, sliced

5 mint leaves

½ of orange, sliced

2 cups of water

Directions:

Divide fruits and mint between two glasses, pour in water, stir until just mixed, and then refrigerate for 2 hours.

Serve straight away.

Nutrition:

Calories: 5.4 Cal

Fat: 0.1 g

Carbs: 1.3 g

Protein: 0.1 g

Fiber: 0.4 g

Chapter 10. Smoothies

310. Chia Berries Smoothie

Cooking time: 5 minutes

Servings: 2

Ingredients

1 cup raspberries, frozen

1 teaspoon ground cardamom

1 1/2 cups almond milk

1/2 cup strawberries, frozen

3 tablespoons chia seeds

Directions:

Add a cup of almond milk into a bowl along with the chia seeds, and then allow to rest for about an hour, until the chia seeds have expanded, and the desired texture turns pudding like.

Put the chia mixture into the blender along with the remaining almond milk, cardamom and the frozen berries. Blitz until combined and smooth.

Pour into chilled glasses and serve.

311. Cucumber Avocado Smoothie

Cooking time: 5 minutes

Servings: 2

Ingredients

1/2 small cucumber

1/2 cup almond milk

2 handfuls fresh baby spinach

1 lemon juiced

1/2 avocado

Directions:

Add all the ingredients for the smoothie to a blender. Blitz until combined and smooth.

Pour into chilled glasses and serve.

312. Hot Pink Smoothie

Cooking time: 5 minutes

Servings: 2

Ingredients

½ cup red berries

¼ teaspoon vanilla extract

1 clementine or tangerine, peeled, chopped

1 tablespoon chia seeds

½ ripe banana, fresh or frozen

2 tablespoons unsalted almond butter, raw or roasted

1 small beet, peeled, chopped

2 tablespoons unsalted almond butter, raw or roasted

1 cup almond milk

Salt, to taste

Directions:

Add all the ingredients for the smoothie to a blender. Blitz until combined and smooth.

Pour into chilled glasses and serve.

313. Maca Caramel Smoothie

Cooking time: 5 minutes

Servings: 2

Ingredients

2 soft Medjool dates, pitted

1/4 cup cold coffee, brewed

1/2 teaspoon vanilla extract

1 handful ice cubes

1/4 cup raw cashews, soaked (4 hours in cold water or 10 minutes in boiling water)

1/2 banana, sliced, frozen

1/4 cup milk, plant-based

1 teaspoon maca powder

1/8 teaspoon salt

Directions:

Add all the ingredients for the smoothie to a blender. Blitz until combined and smooth.

Pour into chilled glasses and serve.

314. Tofu Detox Smoothie

Cooking time: 5 minutes

Servings: 2

Ingredients

1/2 cup bananas, peeled, sliced, frozen

1 cup berries, frozen

1 cup organic spinach or kale

1 cup fruit juice

2 tablespoons silken tofu

1 tablespoon flaxseed meal

Directions:

Add all the ingredients for the smoothie to a blender. Blitz until combined and smooth.

Pour into chilled glasses and serve.

315. Maple Blueberry Shake

Cooking time: 5 minutes

Servings: 2

Ingredients

1/4 cup water

1/2 teaspoon maple extract

1/2 cup cottage cheese, or low-fat yogurt

2 teaspoons flaxseed meal

3 tablespoons vanilla protein powder

1/2 cup frozen blueberries

1/4 teaspoon vanilla extract

Sweetener, to taste

1 handful ice cubes

Directions:

Add all the ingredients for the smoothie to a blender. Blitz until combined and smooth.

Pour into chilled glasses and serve.

316. Valentine Smoothie

Cooking time: 5 minutes

Servings: 2

Ingredients

2 cups soy milk, chilled

2 small figs, fresh

1 teaspoon maca powder

1 tablespoon maple syrup

1/2 teaspoon sweet paprika

1/2 cup cashew nuts

2 tablespoons raw cacao powder

1 cup raspberries, frozen

fresh raspberries, to serve

Directions:

Add all the ingredients for the smoothie to a blender. Blitz until combined and smooth.

Pour into chilled glasses and serve topped with fresh raspberries and a sprinkle of cacao powder.

317. Pina Colada Smoothie

Cooking time: 5 minutes

Servings: 2

Ingredients

13.5 oz. coconut milk

3 bananas peeled, frozen

20 oz. crushed pineapples with juice

Directions:

Add all the ingredients for the smoothie to a blender. Blitz until combined and smooth.

Pour into chilled glasses and serve.

318. Shamrock Smoothie

Servings: 2

Preparation Time: 5 Minutes

Nutrition:

Calories: 39 kcal

Carbs: 5.1g

Fat: 1.8g

Protein: 0.6g

Fiber: 3g

Sugar: 3.1g

INGREDIENTS:

2 cups water

½ cup lettuce

¼ cup pineapple, chopped

½ cup cucumber, peeled and sliced

¼ cup kiwi, peeled and chopped

¼ cup avocado, peeled and pitted

3 tbsp. stevia

DIRECTIONS:

Blend all ingredients together in a blender. Add more or less of what you prefer.

319. The Ultimate Green Smoothie

Servings: 2

Preparation Time: 5 Minutes

Nutrition:

Calories: 104 kcal

Carbs: 8g

Fat: 7.1g

Protein: 2g

Fiber: 4.9g

Sugar: 1.9g

INGREDIENTS:

2 cups spinach

½ avocado, pitted and peeled

½ cucumber

½ cup parsley

1 cup water

Ice cubes (optional

DIRECTIONS:

Blend all ingredients together in a blender. Add more or less of what you prefer.

320. Nutty Green Smoothie

Servings: 2

Preparation Time: 5 Minutes

Nutrition:

Calories: 212 kcal

Carbs: 9.1g

Fat: 16.6g

Protein: 2.9g

Fiber: 4.4g

Sugar: 2.7g

INGREDIENTS:

¼ cup coconut milk

½ avocado, pitted and peeled

½ cup water

½ cup fresh mint

2 tbsp. pistachios

1 tbsp. vanilla extract

2 drops stevia

¼ cup spinach

DIRECTIONS:

Blend all ingredients together in a blender. Add more or less of what you prefer.

A popular favorite! ... and look at the nutritional value of it! A 17g fat content!

321. Coconut Berry Smoothie

Servings: 3

Preparation Time: 5 Minutes

Nutrition:

Calories: 166 kcal

Carbs: 14.7g

Fat: 10.5g

Protein: 3.6g

Fiber: 2.5g

Sugar: 7.5g

INGREDIENTS:

¾ cup frozen blueberries (or your choice of berries

¾ cup almond milk

2 tbsp. ground chia seeds

2 tbsp. coconut oil

3 drops stevia

DIRECTIONS:

Blend all ingredients in a blender in a blender. Add more or less of what you prefer.

322. Fruity Chocolaty Avocado Smoothie

Servings: 2

Preparation Time: 5 Minutes

Nutrition:

Calories: 138 kcal

Carbs: 20.5g

Fat: 4.4g

Protein: 3.0g

Fiber: 3.35g

Sugar: 13g

 INGREDIENTS:

½ cup cashew flavored almond milk

¼ avocado, pitted and peeled

⅓ cup frozen raspberries

1 tbsp. cocoa powder

DIRECTIONS:

Blend all ingredients together in a blender. Add more or less of what you prefer.

323. Chocolate Lover's Smoothie

Servings: 1

Preparation Time: 5 Minutes

Nutrition:

Calories: 232 kcal

Carbs: 9.2g

Fat: 19g

Protein: 3.8g

Fiber: 0.6g

Sugar: 2.9g

INGREDIENTS:

1 tsp. vanilla extract

1 tsp. almond butter

¼ cup coconut milk

¼ cup water

¼ cup cocoa powder

A few dark chocolate chip chunks (optional

DIRECTIONS:

Blend all ingredients together in a blender. Add more or less of what you prefer.

Chapter 11. 21 Day Meal Plan

DAY	BREAKFAST	MAINS	SNACK/DESSERT
1.	Paprika Olives Spread	Mushroom, Lentil, and Barley Stew	Thai Snack Mix
2.	Chives Avocado Mix	Tomato Barley Soup	Zucchini Fritters
3.	Zucchini Pan	Black Beans, Corn, and Yellow Rice	Zucchini Chips
4.	Chili Spinach and Zucchini Pan	Quinoa with Chickpeas and Tomatoes	Quinoa Broccoli Tots
5.	Basil Tomato and Cabbage Bowls	Mushroom Risotto	Spicy Roasted Chickpeas
6.	Spinach and Zucchini Hash	Quinoa and Black Bean Chili	Rosemary Beet Chips
7.	Tomato and Zucchini Fritters	Mexican Stuffed Peppers	Red Salsa
8.	Peppers Casserole	Asparagus Rice Pilaf	Nacho Kale Chips
9.	Spiced Zucchini and Eggplant Bowls	Lentils and Rice with Fried Onions	Tomato Hummus
10.	Spinach and Green Beans Casserole	Vegetable Barley Soup	Rosemary Popcorn

11.	Spinach and Berries Salad	Black Beans and Rice	Marinated Mushrooms
12.	Kale and Broccoli Pan	Portobello Mushroom Stew	Hummus Quesadillas
13.	Leeks Spread	Vegetarian Gumbo	Nacho Cheese Sauce
14.	Eggplant Spread	Root Vegetable Stew	Cinnamon Bananas
15.	Eggplant and Broccoli Casserole	Black Bean and Quinoa Stew	Avocado Tomato Bruschetta
16.	Tomato and Cucumber Salad	Brussel Sprouts Stew	Turmeric Snack Bites
17.	Chia and Coconut Pudding	Fennel and Chickpeas Provençal	Watermelon Pizza
18.	Avocado and Watermelon Salad	Spinach and Cannellini Bean Stew	Pumpkin Cake Pops
19.	Creamy Avocado and Nuts Bowls	Cabbage Stew	Queso Dip
20.	Walnuts and Olives Bowls	Spicy Bean Stew	Nooch Popcorn
21.	Cauliflower Hash	African Peanut Lentil Soup	Honey-Almond Popcorn

Conclusion

As you carefully considered each chapter of this book, we hope that you were able to see the benefits of a Plant-Based Diet. You were able to get the confidence boost you needed to be successful in this transition. You learned exactly what you would be eating and also what you will want to avoid. This hopefully made those trips to the grocery store and market enjoyable. You learned what each category of whole foods you want to keep handy while learning how different whole foods can give you the nutrients you need on a daily basis. You have experienced what it is like to load up your shopping cart with varied delicious fresh foods to make creative and simple meals for the whole family. You learned the importance of avoiding the many common food mistakes that make people quit. You found that this journey is one that can be adjusted to you and your circumstances. That's all there is to know about sticking to it—even when it gets tough. You learned how to create the support and motivation that's needed to keep going. You took on the challenge of adapting your everyday schedule to this wonderful new lifestyle—not letting yourself be worried about what to cook next.

No one can make us make changes in our habits, especially when it comes to eating. Yet, when it is important to get a grip on our physical health, sometimes, a second opinion is warranted. We hope that this book gave you such an opinion.

You learned that a meal plan doesn't have to be scary but an enjoyable adventure that allows you to tap into your creative side in the kitchen. You were able to create an environment that encouraged healthy eating no matter what meal of the day it was—even dessert! You held on to get a good grip not only on setting yourself up for new healthy food choices but also on feeling great as well!

With all of the options and diet choices circling us every day, we hope that you have seen the benefits of choosing a Plant-Based Diet as your gateway to a healthier you!

The next step is to keep going! You learned key steps to making this a lifestyle change—not just a fad. You learned that you aren't perfect—so as long as you put forth every effort, every day, you can take control of your well-being. It will take time to stay balanced with a new eating habit, but the rewards will be worth it!